IMMUNOSCINTIGRAPHY

MONOGRAPHS IN NUCLEAR MEDICINE

A series of books and monographs covering all aspects of nuclear medicine.

Edited by Peter Cox, Rotterdamsch Radio-Therapeutisch Institut

Volume 1
IMMUNOSCINTIGRAPHY
L. Donato and K. Britton

Volume 2
NEW PERSPECTIVES IN NUCLEAR MEDICINE
Edited by P.H. Cox and E. Touja

Additional volumes in preparation

ISSN 0882-6455

IMMUNOSCINTIGRAPHY

Proceedings of the European Symposium on Immunoscintigraphy
held at Saariselka, Finland, 10-12 August 1984

Edited by

L. DONATO
University of Pisa

and

K. BRITTON
St. Bartholomew's Hospital
London

Gordon and Breach Science Publishers
New York · London · Paris · Montreux · Tokyo

Gordon and Breach Science Publishers

P.O. Box 786
Cooper Station
New York, NY 10276
United States of America

P.O. Box 197
London WC2E 9PX
England

58, rue Lhomond
Paris 75005
France

P.O. Box 161
1820 Montreux 2
Switzerland

14-9 Okubo 3-chome
Shinjuku-ku
Tokyo 160
Japan

Library of Congress Cataloging-in-Publication Data
European Symposium on Immunoscintigraphy (1984 : Saariselka, Finland)
   Immunoscintigraphy : proceedings of the European Symposium on Immunoscinigraphy held at Saariselka, Finland, autumn 1984.

   (Monographs in nuclear medicine, ISSN 0882-6455 ; v. 1)
   Includes index.
   1. Cancer— Diagnosis— Congresses. 2. Radioisotope scanning— Congresses. 3. Immunodiagnosis— Congresses. 4. Antibodies, Monoclonal— Diagnostic use— Congresses. 5. Tumor antigens— Analysis— Congresses. I. Donato, L. (Luigi) II. Britton, K. E. (Keith Eric) III. Title. IV. Series. [DNLM: 1. Antibodies, Monoclonal— diagnostic use— congresses. 2. Antigens, Neoplasm— congresses. 3. Isotope Labeling— congresses. 4. Neoplasms— radionuclide imaging— congresses.
   W1 M0568CK v.1 / QZ 241 E895i 1984]
   RC270.E98   1984   616.99'40757   85-17717

Contents

Introduction to the Series

Nuclear medicine is an important and rapidly developing tool for the noninvasive evaluation of pathophysiological processes in vivo. In 1983 we decided to produce the *Radiopharmacy and Radiopharmacology Yearbook* (published by Gordon and Breach Science Publishers, 1st edition 1985) to monitor developments in the basic science of radiopharmacy. It soon became evident that fields of interest could be identified which were worthy of further scrutiny on a broader basis, and from this realization has emerged this series of specialised monographs on selected topics in nuclear medicine. These volumes will be of value not only to the research worker and specialist in nuclear medicine but to all physicians who wish to know how nuclear medical methods can be utilised in their work. The topics that will be covered are far ranging — from the application of monoclonal antibodies, to cancer detection, to the use of nuclear medical techniques in developing countries.

Nuclear medicine is in a constant state of flux. This series will provide a continuous update on topics where significant changes are taking place.

P.H. Cox
C.M. King, Managing Editor

Preface

Cancer is the second most common cause of death in Europe. Its staging and management, the assessment of treatment, and the detection of recurrence remain major requirements for any health service. Trends in this evaluation are on one level directed towards more intensive surgery for staging and debulking the tumour; and at another level towards more detailed and less invasive imaging. In the latter approach, structure still dominates. The site, size, shape, space occupation and relationships of a lesion are determined as a tumour mass and not primarily through its peculiar and particular cancerous nature. The oncogene hypothesis has identified cancer-related genes whose expression in specific cellular and cell surface determinants should one day be identifiable. In the meantime cancer-associated antigens provide the basis for specific imaging and therapy dependant upon the essential characteristics of a tumour and not just on its gross physical properties.

The papers presented at this congress detail the methods available for producing, labelling and using monoclonal antibodies to detect cancer-associated antigens in man and woman. The text provides an overview of the prospects for development in this field. It teaches the preparation and evaluates monoclonal antibodies for their specificity and avidity; the choice of appropriate label and methods of labelling, the techniques and strategies for imaging with these new radiopharmaceuticals. It describes computer analysis of the data obtained and the use of single-photon emission tomography. It details the progress and clinical results in many different cancers to date.

We thank our colleagues for joining us for this meeting within the arctic circle where there was no alternative but that nuclear medicine specialists be exposed to immunology and that immunologists be innoculated with nuclear medicine. We hope that you will be edified by the result.

K. Britton
L. Donato

Acknowledgements

This book is based upon presentations made to a European Symposium on Immunoscintigraphy which was held in Saariselka, Finland, 10-12 August 1984 under the auspices of the ENMS/SNME. The symposium was made possible by organisational and financial support from Sorin Biomedica, Saluggin, Italy. The series editors would like to acknowledge the help of Dr. G.A. Scassellati in screening the manuscripts and Mrs. R. Ripke in preparing the camera-ready copy.

P.H. Cox
C.M. King, Managing Editor

List of First Authors

Britton K.E.
St. Bartholomews Hospital, West Smithfield, London EC1, UK

Buraggi G.L.
Nuclear Medicine Division, Istituto Nazionale Tumori, Milano, Italy

Callegaro L.
Sorin Biomedica, Saluggia (Vercelli) Italy

Chatel J.F.
U.211 Inserm and Centre Rene Gauduchau, Nantes, France

Delaloye B.
Division of Nuclear Medicine, CHUV, 1011 Lausanne, Switzerland

Green A.J.
Cancer Research Campaign Laboratories, Department of Medicinal
Oncology, Charing Cross Hospital, London W6, UK

Goedemans W.T.
Mallinckrodt Diagnostica Holland B.V. Petten, The Netherlands

Hazra D.V.
Nuclear Medicine and RIA Unit, Postgraduate Department of Medicine,
S.M. Medical College, Agra 282005, India

Krohn K.
Institute of Biomedical Sciences, University of Tampere, P.O. Box 607,
33101 Tampere 10, Finland

Mariani G.
CNR Institute of Clinical Physiology, 5th Medical Pathology and Nuclear
Medicine Service of the University of Pisa, Italy

Masi R.
Nuclear Medicine Unit, University of Florence, U.S.L. 10/D Florence,
Italy

Matzku S.
Institute of Nuclear Medicine, German Cancer Research Centre,
Heidelberg, FRG

Oehr P.
Institute of Clinical and Experimental Nuclear Medicine, University of
Bonn, FRG

Pateisky N.
Department of Obstetrics and Gynaecology, University of Vienna, Austria

Perkins A.C.
Department of Medical Physics, Nottingham University Hospital,
Nottingham, UK

Powe J.
Department of Nuclear Medicine, Victoria Hospital, Ontario N6A 4G5,
Canada

Pullano T.G.
Department of Microbiology and Immunology, New York Medical
College, Valhalla NY 10595, USA

Ranki A.
Department of Dermatology, University Central Hospital, University of
Helsinki, Finland

Riva P.
Servizio di Medicina Nucleare e Divisione Dermatologica, Ospedale
Generale Provinciale M. Bufaline, Cesena, Italy

Saccavini J.C.
ORIS-CEA Saclay 91190 Gif/Yvette, France

Siccardi G.S.
Università di Milano, Dipartimento di Biologia e Genetica, Via G.B.
Viotti 5, 20133 Milano, Italy.

Sinn H.
Institute of Nuclear Medicine, German Cancer Research Centre, Im
Neuenheimer Feld 280, D-6900 Heidelberg, FRG

Taylor-Papadimitriou J.
Imperial Cancer Research Fund, P.O. Box 123, Lincoln's Inn Fields,
London WC2A 3PX, UK
Present Address: Royal Postgraduate Medical School, Hammersmith
Hospital, Ducane Road, London W12 0HS, UK

Vihko P.
Department of Clinical Chemistry and Department of Surgery, University
of Oulu, SF-90220 Oulu, Finland

Development of Monoclonal Antibodies useful for localisation of Carcinomas in vivo

Taylor-Papadimitriou J., Griffith A., Epenetos A.[1] and Burcell J.

Imperial Cancer Research Fund,
P.O. Box 123, Lincoln's Inn Fields,
London WC2A 3 PX, U.K.

[1] Present Address:
Royal Postgraduate Medical School,
Hammersmith Hospital,
Ducane Road,
London W12 O.H.S.

INTRODUCTION

The major solid tumours arising in human adults are carcinomas, which develop from epithelial cells. Considerable effort has therefore been put into the development of antibodies reacting with components of the membranes of carcinomas with a view to using them as tools for targeting isotopes in vivo. Many antibodies have been developed which react with antigens expressed by malignant epithelia and some of these have been already tested in the clinic. It is appropriate at this point to assess some of these initial studies primarily to see 1) what are the characteristics of an antibody which is being used with some success and 2) how we can direct our efforts to producing more suitable antibodies. In making such an assessment, it is clear that the antibody cannot be discussed without reference to the antigen, the isotope used for labelling, the topography of the tumour to be localised, and the route of administration. It is also important to remember that there are two main strategic aims in targeting isotopically labelled antibodies to tumours. The first is essentially diagnostic, i.e. to localise tumours and their metastases without surgical intervention and thus improve the management of the cancer patient. The second is investigation of in vivo specificity as a first step in drug targeting. This article will deal primarily with the application of antibodies to tumour localisation, since their efficiency as vehicles for targeting drugs cannot be discussed without defining the drug, isotope or toxin to be targeted.

MONOCLONAL ANTIBODIES USED FOR IN VIVO LOCALISATION OF CARCINOMAS

In attempting to define characteristics of antibodies which might be expected to be effective vehicles for specifically targeting small amounts of an isotope to a tumour it is necessary to also consider the nature of the antigenic site recognised and the antigen–antibody interaction (see Table 1). The antibodies or groups of antibodies which have been investigated in reasonable numbers of patients for localisation of carcinomas are shown in Table 2. Carcinoembryonic antigen (CEA) which is expressed by gastrointestinal and other carcinomas, has been investigated for many years and indeed polyclonal antisera against CEA were tested for tumour localisation before the era of monoclonal antibodies. Antibodies to the human milk fat globule membrane have also been used for several years to characterize cultured

2

mammary cells in culture and tissue sections, but have only recently been applied in patients. The antibody 17.1A is directed to a labile membrane antigen found on gastro-intestinal tumours and on the normal mucosa from which they develop. The antibody 791 T/36 was actually raised against an osteosarcoma, not an epithelial cell line, and appears to localise in the extracellular stromal component of carcinomas (2)

Table 1.

Properties of the antibody-antigen interaction which might lead to effective tumour targeting.

ANTIBODY	ANTIGEN
High avidity for antigenic site	1. Large number of antigenic sites per cell.
Not IgM	2. Low turnover.
Rapid clearance	3. Preferentially expressed on tumour cells.
	4. Not found in high levels in body fluids.
	5. Not lost on metastatic cells.

None of the antibodies referred to in Table 2 can be considered tumour specific since in tissue sections they can be

3

Table 2. Monoclonal antibodies tested for in vivo localisation of carcinomas.

Antibody	Immunising antigen	Antigenic site recognised	General human specificity	Reference
HMFG-2	Human milk fat globule	Carbohydrate antigen on large molecular weight protein(s)	Ovarian and other gynaecological tumours. Breast, some lung and other carcinomas	Epenetos et al., 1982b; Granowska et al., 1984
M8	Human milk fat globule	?	Breast carcinomas	Rainsbury et al., 1983
17.1A	SW1083 (colorectal carcinoma cell line)	?	Gastro-intestinal tract carcinomas	Moldofsky et al., 1983; Shenet et al., 1984; Chatal et al., 1984
19.9	SW116 (colon carcinoma cell line)	Sialylated Le[a]	Gastro-intestinal tract carcinomas; Pancreatic tumours	Chatal et al., 1984
CEA Antibodies	CEA	Protein determinants on CEA	Gastro-intestinal tract carcinomas	Mach et al., 1981; Mach et al., 1983; Chatal et al., 1984
791T/36	791T (osteogenic sarcoma cell line)	72k membrane protein or glycoprotein on 791T cells. Recognises non-epithelial element and any lumenal content of carcinomas.	Gastro-intestinal tract carcinomas; Ovarian carcinomas	Farrands et al., 1982; Armitage et al., 1984; Symond et al., 1984

Table 3. Some examples of monoclonal antibodies reacting with carbohydrate determinants.

Antibody	Immunogen	Antigenic Determinant	Ref.
HMFG-1 HMFG-2	Human milk fat globule	Carbohydrate antigen on large molecular weight molecule (>400k)	Burchell et al., 1983
M18 M39	Human milk fat globule	I(MA) blood group determinant	Gooi et al.,1983
MBr1	MCF-7 cells	carbohydrate	Canevari et al., 1983
19.9	Colorectal cell line	sialylated Le^a	Magnani et al., 1982
Ca1	glycoprotein fraction from MrEp2 cells	Carbohydrate antigen on large molecular weight molecules (390k and 350k)	Ashall et al., 1982
C14/1/46/10	Membrane preparation from human colonic adenoma	Difucosylated Type 2 blood group	Brown et al., 1983

5

seen to react with some normal epithelia. Nevertheless, they have given encouraging results in imaging trials. Here we propose to examine in more detail the properties and specificity of an antibody directed to a component of the human milk fat globule.

ANTIBODIES DIRECTED TO COMPONENTS OF THE HUMAN MILK FAT GLOBULE

The fat globules which are released into the milk during lactation are surrounded by a membrane which is representative of the terminally differentiated mammary epithelial cell. These membranes are easily obtainable from the cream fraction of milk and have been widely used to produce polyclonal antiserum (11) and monoclonal antibodies (see Table 2) which show varying degrees of specificity for epithelial cells in secretory glands or ducts. The most immunogenic component of the human milk fat globule (HMFG) is a large mucin-like glycoprotein (MW >400K) which contains more than 50% carbohydrate (24), and many of the antibodies raised against unfractionated preparations of HMFG are directed to carbonhydrate determinants expressed at various levels on this component. These determinants can also be expressed on components of breast, ovarian and other carcinomas generally derived from secretory epithelia. However, both the size of the component carrying a determinant, and the number of epitopes per molecule may be different in tumours and in the normal secretory cell (7, 8). This almost certainly reflects an abortive processing of the carbohydrate side chains of the secretory mucin by the malignant epithelium which may arise from a changed pattern of glycosyl transferases in the carcinoma. Because of the complexity of expression of the carbohydrate determinants it is possible to find antibodies which, although reacting with the same or similar

6

molecules show a different tissue and tumour specificity. Here we will discuss one antibody (HMFG-2) which is directed to a determinant expressed at a low level on the 400K component produced by the normal secretory mammary cells, but which shows increased expression in breast and other carcinomas (1, 14). It should be noted that this kind of antibody (against a carbohydrate determinant showing increased expression on a large molecular weight membrane component of tumours) has been produced in several laboratories using a variety of tumour cells (or their membranes) as immunogens (4, 5, 6, 17 and see Table 3). The dominance of this type of antibody among those reacting with tumour associated antigens probably reflects both the selective immune response of the mouse and the changed processing of carbohydrate side chains of glycoproteins in human tumours.

SOME FEATURES OF THE ANTIBODY HMFG-2

Within the class of antibodies directed to the large component of HMFG, the antibody HMFG-2 appears to be rather unique in its spectrum of reactivity, in reacting more with malignant than with normal breast epithelium. This may be due to the fact that it was raised in a mouse injected not only with a delipidated preparation of the milk fat globule, but also with cultured growing mammary epithelial cells (26). The mouse was therefore presented with the molecule carrying the antigenic determinant as expressed both on the lactating mammary cell and on a growing non-lactating cell. This could be an important point to remember in trying to raise other antibodies of this type. Antibody HMFG-2 labelled with i^{123} has been used to localise ovarian tumours (14, 18) and is now being used to target lethal doses of ^{131}I by various routes to metastatic carcinoma cells in patients with advanced ovarian cancer and

7

malignant effusions secondary to breast or lung cancer (15). We will discuss the antigen-antibody interaction which has been studied in vitro and in vivo with the aim of defining 1) those features which are advantageous for tumour localisation, 2) those which are not optimal and 3) how we might select for antibodies with improved potential for in vivo use. As indicated previously the antibody can only be considered in relation to other components of the in vivo reaction, i.e. the antigen, the tumour, the isotope and the route of administration.

SPECIFICITY OF REACTION OF HMFG-2

The reaction of an antibody with normal tissues is usually determined by following its reaction with fixed or frozen tissue sections in an enzyme-linked immunohistochemical reaction (e.g. alkaline phosphatase or peroxidase). When looked at in this ways, the antibody HMFG-2 shows a positive reaction with several types of epithelium normally found lining secretory glands or ducts, although liver, the major part of the kidney and the gut, are negative (1, 8). However, in spite of the fact that epithelial cells in tissue sections of normal ovary for example shows a positive reaction, normal ovaries do not show up on a scan in a patient given ^{123}I-HMFG-2. On the other hand, wherever there is disruption of tissue architecture which is the case for inflammatory and benign as well as malignant conditions, localisation of the immunoglobulin in the affected area is detected. This suggests that accessibility of the antigenic site to the antibody plays an important role in determining in vivo specificity. Lining epithelial cells are polarised when in their normal orientation and the HMFG-2 antigen is found on the lumenal surface of the normal cell to which intravenously administered IgG would not have easy access. Access would be increased however when tissue organisation of cellular polarity is lost (3). There is not a great deal of data on binding of antibody to normal and tumour tissues in vivo. Using low doses (400ug-1mg) of antibody, HMFG-2 was found to bind to an ovarian carcinoma but not to normal ovary in patients. However recently, the antibody 17.1A, when given in higher doses was found to bind to normal colonic mucosa as well as to colon carcinoma cells (23). It is important to obtain more data to determine whether the fact that normal tissues are not seen in scans is due to inaccessibility of antigen or to the fact that the antigen is expressed at a reduced level.

AFFINITY OF ANTIBODY FOR ANTIGENIC DETERMINANT(S)

High affinity of the antibody for the antigenic site is an obvious parameter which would be expected to contribute to successful targeting since the antibody should stay bound to the tumour for a long enough period to obtain a definitive scan. This is particularly true if scans are to be done several days after antibody administration. The binding of antibody to the tumour cell however is affected by the nature of the antigenic site as well as the affinity of the antibody for it. Thus, where many epitopes are expressed on the same molecule, bivalent binding of the antibody can occur which results in a much increased avidity. Moreover, the turnover of the molecule expressing the specific determinant will influence the retention of the antibody in the tumour.

The antigenic site recognised by the antibody HMFG-2 is carbohydrate in nature and many epitopes are expressed on a single component which has a low turnover rate. In general this results in a high avidity of antibody for tumour, and when a fairly

9

high dose of ^{131}I-labelled antibody is administered, tumours may be picked up by scanning several weeks after administration (see Figure 1).

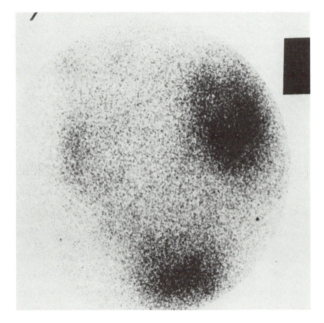

Figure 1.

Abdominal scan taken 4 weeks after intraperitoneal administration of ^{131}I-HMFG-2 for the treatment of ovarian cancer. Note antibody uptake in the large liver metastasis and in a pelvic mass.

However it is important to remember that the avidity can vary from one tumour to another. This has been clearly demonstrated using cultured cell lines (7, 8) and may also be true in vivo. Fig 2a and 2b show the amount of label remaining in tumours in two patients at various times after administration.

TIME COURSE OF ACTIVITY IN RIGHT LUNG
Patient 1.

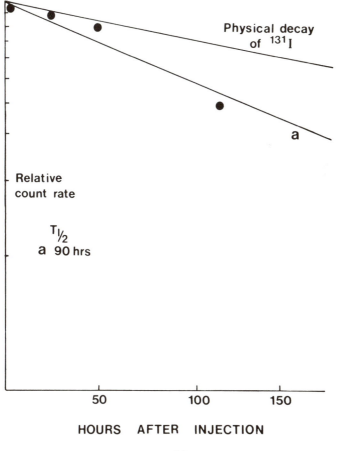

Figure 2a

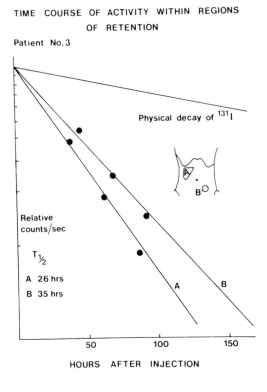

TIME COURSE OF ACTIVITY WITHIN REGIONS
OF RETENTION

Patient No.3

Figure 2b

Figure 2a and 2b.

Decrease in level of tumour-associated ^{131}I–HMFG–2 after intrapleural administration (patient 1 with a pleural effusion secondary to lung adenocarcinoma) and intraperitoneal administration (patient 3 with stage III ovarian cancer).

Tumour-associated radioactivity was determined from scans. As can be seen, the biological half-life of ^{131}I–HMFG–2 is different on tumour targets in the two patients and also different in

12

different tumour areas (A and B) in the same patient.

Clearly label is lost faster in one patient than in the other. Moreover, when two tumours were examined in the same patient the rate of loss of isotope was not identical. Although the clearance of antibody from a tumour site in vivo can be affected by several parameters, it is likely that the avidity of the antibody for the antigenic site is an important one, and will be reflected in the clearance rate. The variation in avidity must be due to subtle differences in the antigenic site recognised, probably related to differences in the size of the component carrying the determinant which as indicated above, can vary, particularly in metastic tumour cells (8).

CLEARANCE OF ANTIBODY

Rapid clearance of antibody remaining after binding to the tumour is obviously desirable to obtain optimum contrast for imaging. However, since it is circulating or bound isotope which gives the background, clearance of antibody will vary with the isotope used. Furthermore, the position of the tumour in relation to the blood pool determines how important total clearance is. The use of ^{123}I-HMFG-2 was first pioneered by Britton and colleagues (14, 18) to localise ovarian tumours allows the maximum contrast to be obtained. However, localisation of say primary breast or lung tumours, using the same labelled antibody is proving to be a much more difficult tast because of their topography. In these cases fast clearance of antibody is essential, if ^{123}I is going to be used, and there is a good case for using $F(ab')_2$ fragments which are cleared much faster than intact antibody. The preparation of antibody fragments is not always straightforward and conditions have to be worked out for each antibody. With HMFG-2, which is an atypical

13

IgG1, very short incubation times are required for optimal yields of the $F(ab')_2$ piece of the molecule. These fragments are now being prepared, but have not yet been tested in vivo (S. Mather, pers. commun.).

If ^{131}I-labelled antibodies are used then it is possible to wait longer for clearance of antibody, and as seen in Figure 1, even four weeks after administration, metastatic ovarian cancer could be detected in a patient given a large amount of ^{131}I-HMFG-2 for therapeutic purposes. It is interesting to note that in this patient the antibody was administered intra-peritoneally to target radioactivity to ovarian cancer cells in ascites. The route of administration is therefore another parameter which affects how much of the antibody gets into the blood and how fast it is cleared from normal tissues and the blood pool.

Undoubtedly it is and will continue to be important to obtain as much data as possible on binding of antibody in vivo and on the pharmacokinetics of clearance. It is possible to follow the amount of labelled antibody in serum and in effusions by separating the fluids on gels and doing an autoradiograph (Figure 3). It is also possible to demonstrate that the circulating antibody still binds to antigen by showing that it binds to specific components expressing the antigen on Western blots (see Figure 4A). Like some other tumour associated antigens that recognised by HMFG-2 can be found circulating in the body fluids (9 and Figure 4B), and the formation of immune complexes could affect both rates and routes of clearance. However, in the case of HMFG-2, the levels of antigen appear to be relatively low, so that some free antibody is available and active, for example 8 hours after administration of only 400 ug (see Figure 4A).

14

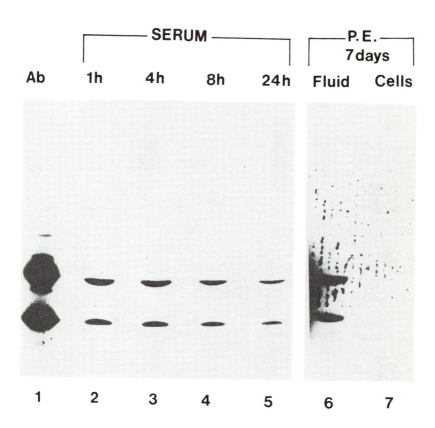

Figure 3.

Detection of labelled antibody in serum and pleural effusion in a patient given ^{131}I-labelled HMFG-2. Samples of serum, effusion fluid or cells isolated from the fluid were run on 5-15% polyacrylamide gradient gels which were subsequently dried and incubated with autoradiographic film. The serum samples were taken at the times indicated and the film was exposed for 5 days. The effusion was collected 7 days after administering the labelled antibody and cells pelleted and washed before extracting for gel

15

B

electrophoresis; in this case the film was exposed for 3 weeks.

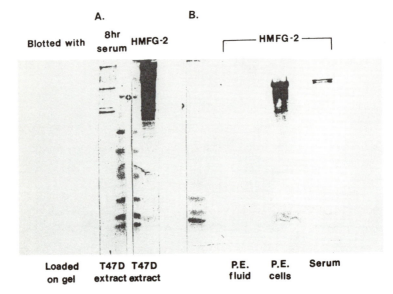

Figure 4.

A. Detection of HMFG-2 antigen in a patient with breast cancer and B. Demonstration of antigen binding HMFG-2 antibody in the serum of a patient given ^{123}I-HMFG-2. A. Extracts of T47D cells were separated on a gel and transferred to nitrocellulose. One track was treated with purified HMFG-2 antibody, and the other with patient's serum, before washing and incubating with peroxidase-linked second antibody followed by substrate. B. Pleural effusion fluid (PE-Fl), patient's serum or an extract of the cancer cells in the pleural effusion (PE-c) were loaded onto a 5–15% polyacrylamide gradient gel and after separation blotted on to nitrocellulose. The blot was stained in an ELISA reaction (7) using a peroxidase linked second antibody and 4-chloronapthol as substrate.

Problems involved in the clearance of indium labelled antibodies include high liver uptake and thus precluding their use for imaging liver metastases. However, indium labelled antibodies appear superior for the imaging of metastases in other body regions.

ANTIBODY CLASS AND SPECIES

For imaging purposes small amounts of antibody are injected and induction of an immune response by the patient may not be a problem. However, if larger amounts are to be given several times, as may be envisaged for therapy, then it would be preferable to use human monoclonals. Clinical trials done so far have however all been with mouse or rat antibodies of the IgG class. Using the classical techniques for production of mouse or rat monoclonals, antibodies of the IgG and IgM class are usually produced, and the larger IgM molecules are unsuitable for in vivo targeting. There has been some suggestion that some mouse IgG2 antibodies recruit host macrophages into a cytotoxic reaction and these although suitable for therapy would be inappropriate vehicles for tumour localisation. HMFG-2 is of the IgG1 class and is therefore suitable for targeting.

DIRECTED PRODUCTION OF ANTIBODIES FOR TUMOUR IMAGING

Although the antibody HMFG-2 has been useful for working out techniques for successful targeting of radioactivity to some carcinomas, it is tumour associated rather than tumour specific – the avidity varies between tumours, and the antigen can be found in body fluids. However, since shotgun type fusions are yielding

17

similar types of antibodies which are against carbohydrate determinants and which may be less useful that HMFG-2, it is worth trying to build on the data we have. We are therefore isolating the components from tumour cells which react with HMFG-2 and using these to obtain other antibodies which 1) may react with a more tumour specific epitope, 2) may have a higher avidity and 3) may not be expressed on the circulating serum component.

REFERENCES

1. Arklie J., Taylor-Papadimitriou J., Bodmer W.F., Egan M. and Millis R. (1981) Differentiation antigens expressed by epithelial cells in the lactating breast are also detectable in breast cancers. Int. J. Cancer 28, 23-29.

2. Armitage N.C., Perkins A.C., Pimm M.V., Farrands P.A., Baldwin R.W. and Hardcastle J.D. (1984) The localization of an anti-tumour monoclonal antibody (791T/36) in gastrointestinal tumours. Br. J. Surg. 71, 407-412.

3. Aronson R.A., Cook S.L. and Roche J.K. (1983) Sensitization to epithelial antigens in chronic mucosal inflammatory desease. 1. Purification, characterization and immune reactivity of murine epithelial cell-associated components (ECAC). J. Immunol. 131, 2796-2804.

4. Ashall F., Bramwell M.E. and Harrid M. (1983) A new marker for human cancer cell. The Ca antigen and the Cal antibody. Lancet 3 July, 1-6.

5. Brockhaus M., Magnani J., Herlyn M., Blaszcyzyk M., Steplewski Z., Koprowski M. and Ginsberg V. (1982) Monoclonal antibodies directed against the sugar sequence of Lacto-N-fucopentaose III are obtained from mice immunized with

human tumours. Arch. Biochem. Biophys. 217, 647–651.

6. Brown A., Feizi T., Gooi M.C., Embleton M.J., Picard J.K. and Baldwin R.W. (1983) A monoclonal antibody against human colonic adenoma recognises difucosylated type-2-blood-group chains. Bioscience Rep. 3, 163–170.

7. Burchell J., Durbin H. and Taylor-Papadimitriou J. (1983) Complexity of expression of antigenic determinants, recognized by monoclonal antibodies HMFG-2 and HMFG-2 in normal and malignant human mammary epithelial cells. J. Immunol. 131, 508–513.

8. Burchell J., Taylor-Papadimitriou J., Granowska M. and Britton K. (1983a) Monoclonal antibodies for successful tumour imaging. Behring Inst. Mitt. 74, 87–93.

9. Burchell J., Wang D. and Taylor-Papadimitriou J. (1984b) Detection of the tumour-associated antigens recognised by the monoclonal antibodies HMFG-1 and 2 in serum from patients with breast cancer. Int. J. Cancer (submitted).

10. Canevari S., Fossat G., Balsari A., Sonnio S. and Colnaghi M. (1983) Immunochemical analysis of the determinant recognised by a monoclonal antibody (MBr1) which specifically binds to human mammary epithelial cells. Cancer Res. 43, 1301–1305.

11. Ceriani R.L., Thompson K., Peterson J.A. and Abraham S. (1977) Surface differentiation antigens of human mammary epithelial cells carried on the human milk fat globule. Proc. Natl. Acad. Sci. U.S.A. 74, 582–586.

12. Chatal J.F., Saccavini J.C., Fumoleau P., Bouillard J.Y., Curtet C., Kremer M., Le Mevel B. and Koprowski H. (1983) Immunoscintigraphy of colon carcinoma. J. Nucl. Med. 25, 307–314.

13. Epenetos A.A., Canti G., Taylor-Papadimitriou J., Curling M. and Bodmer W.F. (1982a). Use of two epithelial-specific

monoclonal antibodies for diagnosis of malignancy in serous effusion. Lancet ii, 1004–1006.

14. Epenetos A.A., Britton K.E., Mather S., Shepherd J., Granowska M., Taylor-Papdimitriou J., Nimmon C., Durbin H., Hawkins L.R., Malpas J.S. and Bodmer W.F. (1982b) Targeting of iodine–123–labelled tumour–associated monoclonal antibodies to ovarian, breast and gastrointestinal tumours. Lancet ii, 999–1004.

15. Epenetos A.A., Courtenay-Luck N., Halnan K.E. Hooker G., Hughes J.M.B., Krausz T., Lambert J., Lavender J.P., MacGregor W.G., McKenzie C.J., Munro A., Myers M.J., Orr J.S., Pearse E.E., Snook D., Webb B., Burchell J., Durbin H., Kemshead J. and Taylor-Papadimitriou J. (1984) Antibody–guided irradiation of malignant lesions: Three cases illustrating a new method of treatment. Lancet June 30, 1441–1443.

16. Farrands P.A., Perkins A.C., Pimm M.V., Hardy J.D., Baldwin R.W. and Hardcastle J.D. (1982) Radioimmunodetection of human colorectal cancers using an antitumour monoclonal antibody Lancet ii, 397–400.

17. Gooi M.C., Uemura K., Edwards P.A., Foster C.S., Pickering N. and Feizi T. (1983) Two mouse hybridoma antibodies against human milk fat globules recognise the I(Ma) antigenic determinant B–D–Gal(1–4) B–D–GlcNAc(1–6). Carbohydrate Res. 120, 293–302.

18. Granowska M., Shepherd J., Britton K.E., Ward B., Mather S., Taylor-Papadimitriou J., Epenetos A.A., Carroll M.J., Nimmon C.C., Hawkins L.A., Flatman W., Horne T. and Bodmer W.F. (1984) Ovarian cancer: Diagnosis using I–123 monoclonal antibody in comparison with surgical findings. Nuclear Med. Commun. (in press).

19. Mach J.P., Buchegger F., Farni M., Ritschard J., Berche

C., Lumbroso J.D., Schreyer M., Girandet C., Accolla R.S. and Carrel S (1981) Use of radiolabelled monoclonal anti-CEA antibodies for the detection of human carcinomas by external photoscanning and tomoscintigraphy. Immunol. Today, Dec. 239–249.

20. Moldofsky P.J., Powe J., Mulhern C.B., Sears H.F., Hammond N.P., Gatenby R.A., Steplewski Z. and Koprowski H. (1983) Imaging with radiolabelled $F(ab')_2$ fragments of monoclonal antibody in patients with gastrointestinal carcinoma. Radiology 149, 549–555.

21. Rainsbury R.M., Ott R.J., Westwood J.H., Kalirai T.S., Coombes R.C., McCready V.R., Neville A.M., Gazet J.C. (1983) Location of metastatic breast carcinoma by a monoclonal antibody chelate labelled with indium–111. Lancet Oct. 22, 934–938.

22. Sears H.F., Mattis J., Herlyn D., Hayry P., Atkinson B., Ernst C., Steplewski Z. and Koprowski H. (1982) Phase I clinical trial of monoclonal antibody in treatment of gastrointestinal tumours. Lancet I, 762–765.

23. Shen J.W., Atkinson B., Koprowski H. and Sears H.F. (1984) Binding of murine immunoglobulin to human tissues after immunotherapy with anticolorectal carcinoma monoclonal antibody. Int. J. Cancer 33, 465–468.

24. Shimizu M. and Yamauchi K. (1983) Isolation and characterization of mucin-like glycoprotein in human milk fat globule membrane. J. Biochem. 91, 515–524.

25. Symonds E.M., Perkins A.C., Pimm M.V., Baldwin R.W., Hardy J.G. and Williams D.A. (1984) Clinical implications for immunoscintigraphy in patients with ovarian malignancy. Br. J. Obstet. Gynaecol. (in press).

26. Taylor-Papadimitriou J., Peterson J., Arklie J.A., Burchell J., Ceriani R.L. and Bodmer W.F. (1981) Monoclonal antibodies to

21

epithelium-specific components of the human milk fat globule membrane: production and reaction with cells of culture. Int. J. Cancer 28, 17-21.

Radiolabelling of monoclonal antibodies for in vivo diagnosis

SACCAVINI J.C., BRUNEAU J., GRZYB J.

ORIS-CEA Saclay 91190 GIF/YVETTE FRANCE

INTRODUCTION

Radioimmunodetection of cancer using radiolabelled antibodies against tumour antigens has recently attracted considerable attention. Although the role of antibody in the detection of cancer was recognized a long time ago, only recently has the possibility to produce large quantities of monoclonal antibodies with a well determined affinity and specificity enabled the use of radiolabelled antibodies on a large scale for the clinical detection of tumours.

Two monoclonal antibodies 19-9 and anti CEA directed against colorectal carcinomas and whose characteristics are described in Table I are in current use in immunoscintigraphy; the clinical results are presented in another paper.

This communication describes the methods used to label these antibodies, the advantages and disadvantages of the different methods, and the effects of the labelling on the antibody molecule, with respect to their physico-chemical and immunological reactivity.

CRITERIA OF CHOICE FOR THE LABELLING OF MONOCLONAL ANTIBODIES

- Choice of useful radioisotopes:-

The selection of radionuclides for radioimmunoimaging is based on the same criteria used to choose nuclides for other studies. A short physical half life and a pure low energy gamma ray (100-300

23

TABLE I : ANTIBODIES USED IN IMMUNOSCINTIGRAPHY

19.9

- IG G 1
- AFFINITY 3.10^7
- ANTIGEN : MONOSIALYLGANGLIOSIDE
- SPECIFIC FOR THE DETECTION OF G.I TUMORS

ANTI - CEA

- IG G 1
- AFFINITY $1.1.10^9$
- ANTIGEN : CEA
- SPECIFIC FOR THE DETECTION OF G.I TUMORS

TABLE II : NUCLIDES USED IN γ IMAGING

RADIONUCLIDE	HALF-LIFE	γ RAY
I^{123}	13.3 HOURS	159 KEV (84 %)
I^{131}	8.05 DAYS	364 KEV (82 %)
IN^{111}	67.5 HOURS	172 KEV 247 KEV (94 %)
GA^{67}	78.1 HOURS	185 KEV (24 %) 300 KEV (16 %)
TC^{99M}	6 HOURS	140 KEV (88 %)

TABLE 111

LABELLING THE 19.9 F(AB')2 WITH L131
BY THE CHLORAMINE T METHOD

Quantity Chloramine T	Ratio AB/CT	Reaction Time	Immunoreactivity
100 uG	10	3-min	42%
100 uG	10	1-min	65%
50 uG	20	3-min	41%
50 uG	20	1-min	70%

AB – antibody

CT – chloramine T

KeV) are suitable, first to enable a good detection by the gamma camera, and secondly to deliver minimum radiation dose to the patient.

The radionuclides easily available for in vivo diagnostic use are limited. The nuclides commonly used in imaging are shown in Table II together with their physical properties.

- CHOICE OF THE LABELLING TECHNIQUE:-
  - the labelling should be quick and easy to perform;
  - the labelling yield and the specific activity should be high
  - The biological and immunological properties of the should be preserved;
  - The bond between radionuclide and antibody should be sufficiently firm.

LABELLING WITH IODINE

For radioiodination of the antibodies many methods are available. But, considering the criteria described earlier only three methods were investigated: the use of oxidizing agents (chloramine T), iodogen and lactoperoxidase.

The lactoperoxidase (1) method is enzymatic, so it is very mild, and the protein denaturation is minimal. But the labelling is long and the yield of incorporation of iodine is not very high; moreover the purification step is long because lactoperoxidase has to be separated from the labelled antibody.

The chloramine T (2) method is quick, easy to perform and a very high specific activity and labelling yield are obtained. But chloramine T is a highly reactive agent and can cause denaturation and polymerisation of proteins. Therefore the quantity of chloramine T and the time of reaction are very important factors in radioiodination as is shown in the labelling of 19-9 $F(ab')_2$ antibody (Table III).

The iodogen (3) method is easy to perform and a very high

26

TABLE lV

Comparison between the three techniques

Technique	Antibody	Yield of incorporation	Immunoreactivity
Chloramine T	19.9F(ab')2	88 %	72 %
Lactoper-oxidase	"	65 %	83 %
Iodogen	"	91 %	85 %
Chloramine T	Anti CEA	58 %	70 %
Lactoper-oxidase	"	25 %	68 %
Iodogen	"	78 %	77 %

specific activity and labelling yield are obtained. Iodogen is very poorly soluble in water; the reaction occurs in a solid phase, thus denaturation of protein is minimal and purification is easily achieved with a very small anionic exchange column. But the reaction time depends on the antibody and must be studied in each case (see figures 1 and 2 relative to the labelling of 19–9 and anti CEA antibodies).

In Table IV the three methods are compared for labelling of the two antibodies. The results obtained show the advantage of the iodogen method. This technique is easy to perform and offers a high labelling yield, comparable to that obtained with chloramine T and an immunoreactivity comparable to that obtained with lactoperoxidase.

These two antibodies are now routinely labelled via the iodogen method and the general process of labelling and purification is described in Table V.

LABELLING WITH METALLIC RADIONUCLIDES

For labelling with these radionuclides two points have to be considered:

- direct labelling is in many cases not possible, because Nuclides have no affinity for proteins;
- when direct labelling is possible, the stability constant is generally too weak and some transchelation with other plasma proteins occurs in vivo.

So, for labelling, bifunctional chelating agents are used, which form stable protein conjugates and bind metal ions very tightly.

Chelating agents such as E.D.T.A. and D.T.P.A. are known to form strong complexes and have been widely used to bind metal ions to a variety of simple and complex organic molecules.

The two antibodies 19–9 and anti CEA were labelled with indium or gallium via D.T.P.A.

Two reactions were considered to conjugate D.T.P.A. to the

28

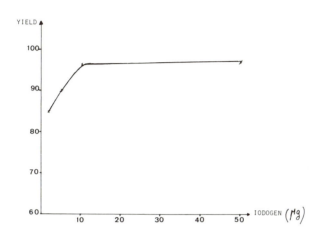

Fig. 1. Efficiency of 19-9 antibody labelling with I^{131} as a function of the iodogen quantity (reaction time 10 min).

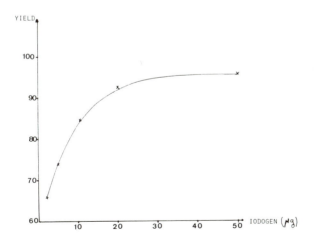

Fig. 2. Efficiency of anti CEA antibody labelling with I^{131} as a function of the iodogen quantity (reaction time 10 min).

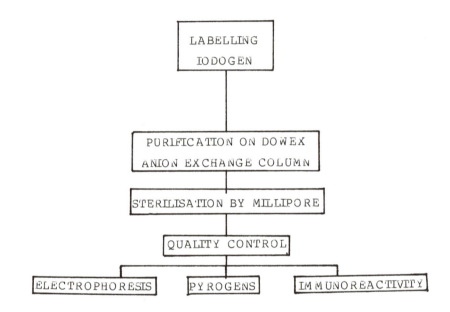

Table V : General process of labelling and purification
of antibodies using Iodine.

Table VI : Methods used to conjugate DTPA

DOUBLE ANHYDRIDE

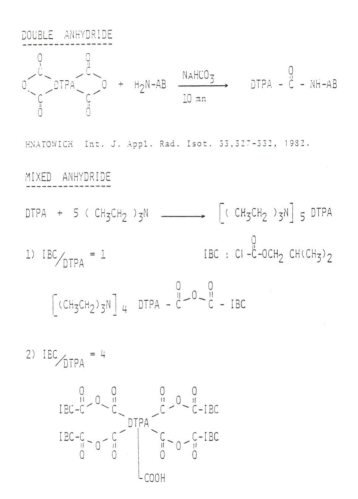

HNATOWICH   Int. J. Appl. Rad. Isot. 33,327-332, 1982.

MIXED ANHYDRIDE

$DTPA + 5 (CH_3CH_2)_3N \longrightarrow \left[(CH_3CH_2)_3N \right]_5 DTPA$

1) $IBC/_{DTPA} = 1$ $IBC : Cl-\overset{O}{\overset{\|}{C}}-OCH_2 CH(CH_3)_2$

$\left[(CH_3CH_2)_3N \right]_4 DTPA - \overset{O}{\overset{\|}{C}} - O - \overset{O}{\overset{\|}{C}} - IBC$

2) $IBC/_{DTPA} = 4$

KREJCAREK   Biophys. Res. Com. 77 (2), 581-585, 1977.

- the bicyclic anhydride prepared following the protocol described by Hnatowich (4). It is a reaction of acylation between the anhydride groups and amino groups of the proteins. The conjugation is achieved in ten minutes in bicarbonate buffer pH 8.

- The mixed anhydride prepared following the protocol described by Krejcarek (5). The mixed anyhydride is produced in situ just before the conjugation.

The coupling is also achieved in bicarbonate buffer pH 8, but the reaction time is about one hour at room temperature.

For each method the influence of the ratio DTPA anhydride/antibody on the formation of dimeric form and on the immunoreactivity of the antibody was studied. The rate production of the dimeric form was determined by uv. detection after separation by H.P.L.C. on a T.S.K. 3000 column.

- METHOD OF THE MIXED ANHYDRIDE:-

For the ratio DTPA/IBC 1:1, the anhydride produced remains low; but by raising the ratio DTPA/IBC from 1:1 to 1:4 the quantity of anhydride produced is highly increased. In Table VII, the results obtained show that the rate of production of the dimeric form is related to the quantity of anhydride; and the presence of dimeric form results in a decrease of the immunoreactivity of the antibody.

- METHOD OF DOUBLE ANHYDRIDE:-

The efficiency of the method, and the amount of D.T.P.A. effectively conjugated to the proteins was measured after labelling with indium.

In Table VIII the results obtained show that the efficiency of

32

TABLE Vll

Effect of conjugation of DTPA on antibody activity (method of the mixed anhydride)

DTPA/Ab Molar Ratio	DTPA/L.B.C Molar Ratio	Dimeric Form U.V.Determination	% Active Antibody
100	1 : 1	−	75%
100	1 : 2	−	73%
100	1 : 3	10–15 %	64%
100	1 : 4	30–40 %	43%

TABLE Vlll

Effect of conjugation of DTPA on antibody Binding Activity (double anhydride method)

Anhydride/Ab Molar Ratio	No of DTPA Incorporated	Dimeric Form U.V Determination	% Active Antibody
2 .5	1	−	74%
5	1.8	15–20%	69%
10	5	27–33%	64%
20	7.6	35–40%	53%

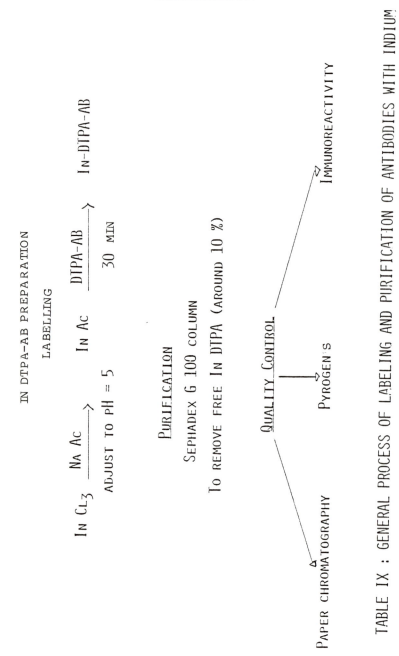

TABLE IX : GENERAL PROCESS OF LABELING AND PURIFICATION OF ANTIBODIES WITH INDIUM

the method is about 40 %. As the amount of D.T.P.A. linked to the proteins increases, the formation of dimeric form rises and results in a decrease in the immunoreactivity of the antibody.

- Conclusion:-

It has been found that the D.T.P.A. anhydride efficiently conjugates antibodies, but may decrease antigen binding if the extent of conjugation is too high.

Since small quantities of chelated proteins are used, it is especially important to keep all solutions free of contaminating metals. So it is preferable to use the method of Hnatwich to conjugate DTPA with antibodies because the step of purification consists of a simple gel chromatography without long dialysis.

For the labelling with indium or gallium, acetate complexes are first produced then the metal ions exchange easily from the acetate to protein-bound D.T.P.A. at pH 5.5.

Table IX gives the general process of production on indium - D.T.P.A. - antibody.

CONCLUSION

Dehalogenation is a major problem when antibodies are labelled with isotopes of iodine; about fifty per cent of the radioiodine are removed from the protein within 48 hours. The result of this dehalogenation is a rapid clearance of the tracer from various organs and possibly from the tumour.

Indium or gallium nuclides have many favourable properties, the half-life matches well with the maximum tumour concentration, and these compounds are stable when bifunctionally chelated on to antibody. But, with these products, about twenty per cent of the injected dose is accumulated in the liver, which is a great disadvantage for the visualisation of liver metastasis.

Therefore for the labelling of antibodies the choice of the

nuclide depends on what you want to do, and what you want to
see in vivo.

BIBLIOGRAPHY

(1) Marchalonis
     Biochem J., 113, 299–305, 1969.

(2) Greenwood F.C., Hunter W.H.
     Biochem. J., 89, 114–123, 1963.

(3) Fraker P.J., Speck J.C.
     Biochem. and biophys, Res. Comm., 80, (4), 849–857,, 1978.

(4) Hnatowich D.S., Layne W.W., Chilos R.L.
     Int. J. Appl. Rad. Isot., 33, 327–332, 1982.

(5) Krejcarek G.E., Tucker K.L.
     Biochem. Biophys, Res. Comm. 77, (2), 581–585, 1977.

Labelling and purification procedures

H. SINN

Institute of Nuclear Medicine, German Cancer Research Centre, Im Neuenheimer Feld 280, D-6900 Heidelberg, FRG.

According to the present state of knowledge, iodine labelling procedures in aqueous solutions can be separated into three groups:

1. Nucleophilic isotope or halogen exchange with iodide.
2. Electrophilic isotope or halogen exchange with iodine.
3. Electrophilic hydrogen substitution in aromatic ring systems by iodine.

The labelling mechanisms 1. and 2. presume the existence of stable halogen containing molecules. There is no or only a minor change in the characteristics of the starting material. The third type of reaction, which is basically a direct halogenation, can be used for tagging a variety of substances. It is of great importance since very sensitive compounds such as proteins can be labelled in this way. If the procedure is not carried out with very great care, the tagging may be accompanied by serious alterations to the molecule.

While the nucleophilic iodine exchange has been used for more than 20 years, especially for production of radioiodine labelled ortho-iodo-hippuric acid (3,8,10,11), the exchange, consciously following the electrophilic mechanism is rarely done (1,2,7,9). In spite of the extended knowledge of nucleophilic exchange reactions, some problems arose when I-123 and I-121 were available. The fairly short physical half lives, of 13 hrs and 2 hrs respectively, made the required minimal reaction time a predominant factor. Alterations in activity concentrations and variable impurities such as iodate and periodate created additional problems.

We found that the problem of iodate and periodate contamination was a minor one. It does not exist if the reaction temperature is raised above 155°C. Low and alterable activity concentrations were a more serious barrier to a clean, fast, and efficient labelling method.

Extended trials resulted in the use of a double chambered reaction vial (Fig.1.).

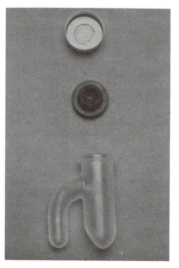

FIGURE 1. Reaction vial for nucleophilic radioiodine labelling procedures. A water binding agent (e.g. Calcium chloride) is placed in the side chamber whereas radioiodine and the organic compound are placed together in the main chamber.

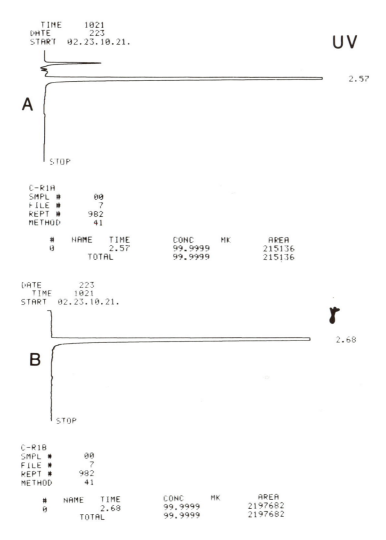

FIGURE 2 HPLC records of a normal control chromatogram of radioiodine labelled ortho-iodo-hippuric acid. Upper part (A) UV record, lower part (B) simultaneously registered data of the gamma detector.

If the delivered I-123 concentrations are low, i.e. below 10 mCi/200 ul, the use of a triple chambered reaction vial reduces problems considerably (Fig.3).

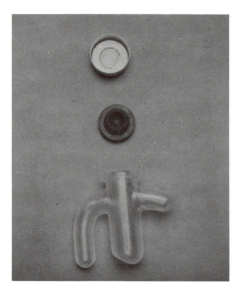

FIGURE 3   Reaction vial for electrophilic radioiodine labelling procedures. A water binding agent (e.g Calcium chloride) is placed in the larger side chamber whereas the oxidizing agent is in the smaller one. Radioiodine and the organic compound are placed in the middle chamber.

One side chamber contains $CaCl_2$ as the water binding agent while the other is loaded with $HAuCl_4$. Radioiodine and the inactive organic compound are brought together in the middle chamber. At the end of the reaction, free iodine and $HAuCl_4$ are separated together in a single passage on an anion exchange resin (e.g. Bio Rad AG 1x8). The average yield is about 80%. The radiochemical purity approaches 100%.

The reaction components, radioiodine and the carrier molecule e.g. ortho-iodo-hippuric acid (oIH), are placed together in the main chamber. A water binding agent ($CaCl_2$) is placed in the side chamber. During the heating period water is withdrawn from the reaction solution. In this way the iodine exchange is done in parallel with the required volume reduction without any delay. With a reaction time of about 12 min an average labelling yield of 99.7% is achieved (Fig.2).

High Performance Liquid Chromatography, sometimes demonstrates two impurities: about 0.1% of iodide and up to 0.3% of ortho-iodo-benzoic acid.

Substances which can be labelled adequately are:

Amidotrizoic Acid

Iothalamic Acid

Iodoxamic Acid

17-I-Heptadecanoic Acid

Lipiodol

The second type of reaction, the electrophilic exchange is used primarily for those chemical compounds which react better under electrophilic exchange conditions than with the nucleophilic exchange. Metrizamide and Iopamidol belong to this group as well as isopropyl-iodo-amphetamine and meta-iodo-benzylguanidine. When tetra-chloro-gold acid ($HAuCl_4$)is used as the iodine producing agent, the required reaction parameters are:

reaction temperature: below 130°

reaction time: 25 min.

The anion exchange resin column is lead shielded and in truth a modified dry column technetium generator. We use the same system for purification of radioiodine labelled oIH and other compounds listed under the nucleophilic reaction. In this case we use silver chloride (AgCl) as the iodine trapping material. The cleansing capacity of this system is demonstrated in Fig. 4. To demonstrate the effectiveness of the procedure, we added 4% of radioiodide to a clean solution of OIH. A single passage over the silver chloride column separated the unbound iodine quantitatively.

In contrast to the electrophilic exchange reactions, where the purification step which separated the oxidizing agent is an essential part of the procedure, we use the cleansing system in the nucleophilic reactions only as a security factor. In a normal running reaction with 0.1% of unbound iodine we do not need a purification. A different and important aspect is the necessity to clean stock solutions of I-131 labelled compounds every day and separate unbound iodine produced by radiolysis.

The third labelling mechanism, the electrophilic hydrogen substition is known in nuclear medicine since Fine published an indirect, and Keston a direct method in 1944 for tagging proteins with radioiodine (4,5). In the meantime a large number of papers were published on this topic. Direct labelling methods are presented, as are indirect ones. The advantages or disadvantages of different oxidizing agents such as hydrogen peroxide, iodine chloride, Chloramine—T, Iodogen etc. were discussed as well as one or two phase reactions. Time intervals of a few seconds to several hours are reported as being optimal, as well as pH ranges from 7.0 to 13. However, all methods show conformation in one respect that at the end of the reaction they all need a purification step. This is to separate unbound iodine, denaturated protein and perioxidase

42

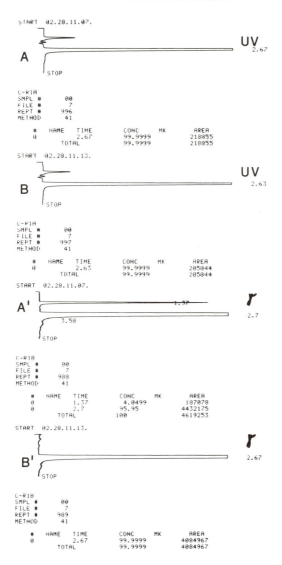

FIGURE 4 HPLC records of radioiodine labelled ortho-iodo-hippuric acid (oIH). A and A' show the corresponding UV and gamma records of an oIH contaminated with 4% of iodide. B an B' show the corresponding UV and gamma records of the same preparation after a single passage through a silver chloride column

43

or Chloramine–T. In most cases this purification is done by gel chromatography, sometimes by dialysis.

As long as the activities handled are less than 3 mCi there is no problem. Problems, however, arise when the requested activities rise to 30 mCi or more. This level is necessary for patients undergoing radiotherapy with I-131 labelled monoclonal antibodies. Starting with I-131 and monoclonal antibodies and considering the reported relatively low yields of labelled proteins, this approach would result in a high priced end product. The personnel handling these high activities will have a high irradiation exposure. Last but not least, the amount of radioactive waste, volume as well as activity level, is an important factor influencing the costs of a radioiodine labelled compound. With this in mind we sought to find a protein labelling procedure which did not require a purification step.

We were convinced that N–bromo–succinimide (NBS) would be the optimal agent to produce the required iodonium ion. A literature search pointed to an absolutely opposite result (12). Compared to chloramines as Chloramine–T the labelling efficiencies with NBS were moderate. This was disappointing, but we started our own trials. In the beginning NBS was used in quantities comparable to those of Chloramine–T. We used NBS in a range of 20 to 50 ug per mCi radioiodine together with 300 to 500 ug of protein. The results were not encouraging. This changed considerably when the quantity of NBS was reduced stepwise. Presently we achieve labelling yields of 98% with 1.2 ug of NBS (= 0.5 ug Br$^+$) per mCi I-131. A trial with 5 mg protein, 15 mCi I-123 and only 10 ug NBS, this means 0.7 ug NBS/mCi, showed that 8% of iodine remained unbound (Fig.5).

The percentage of parallel bromine incorporation with the iodine–tagging can be easily evaluated by replacing I-131 with carrier free Br-77 (Fig.6). The comparison of areas in the TLC-record shows that only 8–10% of the bromine atoms are taken up by the protein corresponding to 0.05 ug of bromine. The use of such tiny quantities of the oxidizing agent Br^+ (0.5 ug/mCi I-131), which has additionally a lower oxidation power than Cl^+ implies two things:

1. A markedly reduced amount of sodium meta bisulphite to stop the reaction.

2. The prevention of denaturation of the relevant protein.

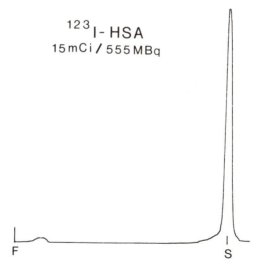

^{123}I- HSA
15mCi / 555MBq

F

S

FIGURE 5 Thin layer chromatogram of a 1–123 labelled HSA
S = starting point, F = front
Rf values: ^{123}I-HSA: 0.0 ^{123}I- : 0.9

45

This prevention of protein denaturation could be proven with an animal experiment. A non-purified I-131-RSA was applied to rats intraveneously. At different time intervals blood samples were taken over a period of 10 days. The resulting curve (fig.7) was identical to results published by McFarlane in 1956 using a C-14 and I-131 double labelled and purified protein.

^{77}Br - BSA

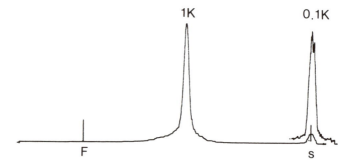

FIGURE 6   Thin layer chromatogram of a Br-77 HSA control labelling. S = starting point; F = front line; Rf values: ^{77}Br-HSA : 0.0; ^{77}Br- : 0.55 sensitivity of rate meter: 1 K and 0.1 K.

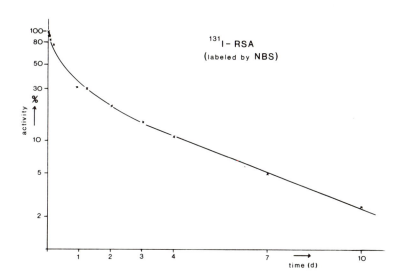

FIGURE 7   Activty levels after the injection of an unpurified
radioiodine labelled RSA into rats.

SUMMARY

Exchange labelling procedures can be done following:

1. A nucleophilic reaction mechanism
2. An electrophilic reaction mechanism

        Both   procedures   are   a   minimum   of   necessary
handling, combined with a maximum of efficiency and security
using special reaction vials.

47

C

Protein labelling can be done approximately quantitatively, if NBS, used in the same amounts as radioiodine, is brought into the reaction. The elimination of purification steps reduces the irradiation exposure of the personnel as well as the costs of the respective products.

LITERATURE

1. Anghiliere, L.I.: A Simplified Method for Preparation High Specific Activity I^{131}-Labelled Hippuran
Int. J. Appl. Radiat. Isotopes 15, 95 (1964)
2. Belkas, E.P., E.Hiotllis and C. Dassiou: Hippuran-^{131}I; Preparation and Purity Control
Int. J. Appl. Radiat. Isotopes 26, 629 (1975)
3. Elias, H., Ch. Arnold and G. Kloss: Preparation of ^{131}I-Labelled m-Jodohippuric Acid and its Behaviour in Kidney Function Studies Compared to o-Jodohippuric Acid
Int. J. Appl. Radiat. Isotopes 24, 463 (1973)
4. Fine, J., and A.M. Seligman: Traumatic Shock. VII. A Study of the Problem of the "Lost Plasma" in Hemorrhagic, Tourniquet and Burn Shock by the Use of Radioactive Jodoplasma-Protein
J. Clin. Invest. 23, 720 (1944)
5. Keston, A.S.: The Schradinger Enzyme in Biological Iodinations
J. Biol. Chem. 153, 335 (1944)
6. McFarlane, A.S.: Labelling of plasma proteins with radioactive iodine
Biochem. J. 62, 135 (1956)
7. Mills, S.L.: Rapid Synthesis of ^{123}J-Labelled Iodinated Contrast Media by "Kit"-Type Labelling Procedure

48

Int. J. Appl. Radiat. Isotopes 33, 467 (1982)

8. Scheer, K.E., W. Maier-Borst: Die Darstellung von ^{131}J-Ortho-Jodhippursaure (Hippuran) durch Austauschmarkierung.

Nucl. Med. (Stuttgart) 2, 163 (1962)

9. Sharma, H.L., and A.G. Smith: Labelling Metrizamide (Amipaque) with Iodine-125

Acta Radiol. Diagnosis 20, 289 (1979)

10. Sinn, H., W.Maier-Borst, H.Elias: An Efficient Method for Routine Production of o-Jodohippuric Acid Labelled with ^{131}I, ^{125}I or ^{123}I

Int. J. Appl. Radiat. Isotopes 28, 809 (1977)

11. Thakur, M.L., B.M. Chauser; The Preparation of Iodine-123 Labelled Sodium Ortho-Iodo-Hippurate and its Clearance by the Rat Kidney.

12. Youfeng, H., H.H. Coenen, G. Petzold, and G. Stocklin: A Comparative Study of Radiaiodination of Simple Aromatic Compounds via N-Halosuccininides and Chloramine-T in TFAA.

J.Label. Compds. 19, 807 (1982)

Experience with 123 I-Labelled monoclonal antibodies

Britton K.E., Granowska M., Mather S. & Nimmon C.C.
St. Bartholomew's Hospital, West Smithfield, London E.C.1.

Nuclear Medicine is based on the development of new radiopharmaceuticals. Radionuclide labelled antibodies are a new class of radiopharmaceutical and their future success will depend on an understanding of the physical requirements for a good imaging technique so that the optimal compromise between conflicting features may be obtained.

For static imaging the key requirement is a high count rate delivered from the tissue of interest. In order to obtain this the choice of radionuclide is of prime importance. The emitted gamma ray must be sufficiently energetic so that tissue absorption does not reduce sensitivity too much but not so energetic that it passes through the thin crystal of the gamma camera. The ideal energy of a gamma ray to interact efficiently with the crystal of the gamma camera is between 100 and 200 KeV and the nearer to the top end of this scale, the less the tissue absorption. In order to obtain a high count rate, the radionuclides should have a short half life so that a large dose may be administered to the patient and yet give a low radiation exposure, since the absorbed dose depends on the activity received integrated over time. The time course of the uptake of the pharmaceutical is also crucial to selection of the radionuclide since if its half life is too short, the count rate would be inadequate at the time of maximum uptake. To reduce radiation exposure to the patient it is also important that the radionuclide is free of beta particle radiation. A high count rate is essential for the detection of small lesions, thus a radioactive pin head is detectable if it contains enough activity. It will be presented on an image as an area of uptake much larger than its physical size, because the resolution of the modern camera is of the order of 1.5 cm at depth. Only over 2 cm diameter lesions, is there a rough correspondence between image size and lesion size. Thus it should be appreciated that primary detection depends importantly on the count rate obtained from the object of interest, and this in turn is determined by the choice of radionuclide label if the characteristics of the antibody in terms of avidity, specificity and uptake are the same whatever the label.

The second requirement for detection is the Signal to noise ratio; that is the count rate in the object of interest in relation to the count rate in its environment. The optimisation of this ratio depends primarily on the selectivity of the radiopharmaceutical for the object of interest as compared with its background. Thus the liver is easily visualised virtually free of tissue background using $^{99}Tc^m$ Sn colloid, because over 70 % of the injected activity is in the organ of interest within a few minutes. When the radiopharmceutical is a labelled antibody and the object of interest a tumour, then the signal to noise ratio will depend on the avidity of the antibody for the tumour and on its specificity. Since the uptake in man of currently available labelled antibodies is a low percentage of the amount injected – in the order of 1 % and the highest recorded uptake being of the order of 7 % – then the differential rates of clearance of the antibody from the tumour and from its environment become important. Two approaches are

52

made to this situation. The first is to increase the clearance rate of the antibody itself by the use of antibody fragments[1]. It is crucial with this approach that the amount of antibody taken up by the tumour is not reduced either through reduction in avidity of the fragment as compared to the whole antibody or through any reduction in residence time of the antibody for example through more rapid metabolism. The reduction in size of the antibody when presented to the tumour as an active fragment may have an advantage of easier penetration into the tumour. For the Fab fragment approach to make a significant contribution to tumour detection, the clearance rate should be improved by a factor of four times. An alternative approach is to use the injection of a second antibody, either free or liposome bound[2], to pull the targetting antibody out of the circulation.

Since the rate of clearance of the antibody bound to the tumour is much slower than its rate of clearance from the tissue environment, the use of a long half life label such as ^{131}I will lead to an improvement in signal to noise ratio over time as compared with a shorter lived label such as ^{123}I or ^{111}In. However it cannot be overstressed that such an approach leads to low count rates in the target and the background. Since the noise due to poisson statistics in gamma ray detection depends on the square root of the count rate, the lower the count rate, the disproportionately higher is the noise. Thus at 10.000 cpm, the noise is 100 cpm that is 1% of the counts recorded whereas at 100 cpm the noise is 10 cpm that is 10% of the counts recorded. This primary type of degradation of the signal severely reduces tumour detectability. This is discussed below. The necessary requirement for improving the signal to noise ratio is through an increase in the specificity, avidity and therefore uptake of the antibody and

53

its attached label rather than concentrating on improving the rate of clearance from the tissue environment.

The radionuclides available for labelling antibodies may be considered and their advantages and disadvantages are summarised in Table I. ^{123}I best fits the criteria set out previously because the highest count rate for the lowest absorbed radiation dose can be obtained per unit of activity administered. This is because ^{123}I has a high abundance of gamma rays of an energy ideal for the gamma camera and this with its short half life and the use of a low energy collimator with thin septa allows a count rate to be obtained which is about one hundred times that obtained with ^{131}I for the same administered activity. Its availability however is limited, usually once weekly, and in lower specific activity than ^{131}I. For labelling, added carrier stable iodine is necessary to push the reaction to completion, thus synthesis of the labelled antibody is a little more difficult than with ^{131}I. It costs 15 Pounds Sterling per mCi (40 MBq) delivered from the Atomic Energy Research Establishment, Harwell. 5 mCi (200 MBq) are used for labelling per study, giving an injectate of labelled antibody containing about 3-4 mCi (120-160 MBq) and a total cost of 75 Pounds for the radionuclide. The labellling technique is described below.

^{131}I has the disadvantage of producing beta rays which give 80% of the radiation due to this radionuclide. The long half life means also that only a relatively small amount of activity should be given. In radiation dosimetry terms, the injection of 1-2 mCi (40-80 MBq) ^{131}I labelled antibody is much too high for diagnostic use. For example 4 mCi free ^{131}I is often used as therapy dose for thyrotoxicosis. While it may be argued that high absorbed doses are acceptable in patients with known cancer, likely to receive radiotherapy or chemotherapy, the situation is different when such studies are to be used in more general diagnostic role. The high energy penetrates the thin crystal of the modern gamma camera so the efficiency of count collection is poor and a medium energy collimator with thick septa has to be used which degrades sensitivity. However the ready availability, cheapness, and ease of labelling with ^{131}I commend it as the label with which new studies are commenced.

A general advantage of the radioisotopes of iodine is that the labelling of antibodies with iodine has been routine in the field of radioimmunoassay. In order to label the antibody at a site away from the active centre so as not to affect its immunospecificity a 1:1 Iodine to antibody molar radio is recommended. The use of radio-iodine has some disadvantages. The patient requires loading with stable iodine, for example, potassium iodide 60 mg daily from the day before and for three days after the study for ^{123}I and for two weeks after ^{131}I. It is evident from animal studies that the iodine label attached to antibody bound to tumour does not come off. The in vivo metabolism of iodine labelled antibody not bound to tumour is relatively rapid and about 20% free iodine is liberated in 24 hours. Whether the iodine is bound or free in blood or tissue other than the cancer, it all contributes to the background 'noise' against which the signal from the cancer has to be determined.

^{111}I Indium has an excellent gamma ray energy 0.17 MeV for the gamma camera, but unfortunately it has a gamma ray of higher energy 0.25 MeV which necessitates the use of a medium energy collimator to prevent septal penetration. The heavier collimator reduces sensitivity and resolution as compared to the lighter one used for ^{123}I and ^{99}Tc^{m}. However its 67 hour half life has the potential commercial advantage that there would be time for a manufacturer to label, undertake quality control, package and distribute ready labelled antibody to centres undertaking radioimmunoscintigraphy. The labelling procedure is more complex and requires the use of bifunctional chelate, one end of which binds the Indium and the other binds the protein[3,4]. The cyclic anhydride of diethylene triamine penta acetate, DTPA, is a satisfactory chelate for this purpose. The cost of the ^{111}In chloride for labelling antibody in house is high,97 Pounds Sterling per dated 2 mCi (80 MBq) vial which contains more activity than this when delivered. 6 mCi starting material per patient dose is required (200 Pounds) ^{111}In labelled antibody is less rapidly metabolised in the body, about 5% per 24 hours than radio-iodine labelled antibody. However a higher than expected liver uptake of the ^{111}In labelled antibody may be seen. Free ^{111}In is bound to plasma transferrin and ^{111}In DTPA is excreted in the urine.

^{99}Tc^m Technetium is the standard radionuclide of nuclear medicine being generator produced on site, but it has two major disadvantages in this context. It is particularly difficult to label biologically active proteins in a way to that they remain stable in vivo for 24 hours and its short half life of six hours means that too little activity is present at the time of maximum antibody uptake which is between 12-24 hours. In conclusion for the buying in of manufactured labelled antibody the use of ^{111}In is required, but for in house labelling of antibody ^{123}I has advantages over ^{111}I in terms of cost, sensitivity and resolution but is less widely available. However if the rate of uptake of the antibody by the tumour is thought not to reach a maximum until 2 days after administration which is usual, then the longer half life ^{111}In has an advantage in enabling delayed imaging at 48 hours. ^{123}I imaging is most effective up to 24 hours.

Technique of labelling with ^{123}I

^{123}I Iodine is produced by the Atomic Energy Research Establishment, Harwell, using a high energy cyclotron so that the product ^{123}I is free of ^{124}I and contains less than 0.05% ^{125}I. It is available throughout Europe on a Wednesday morning. It is dissolved in sodium Hydroxide, dispensed into sterile vials and may be dried. Iodogen (Tetrachlorodi-phenylglycoluril-Pierce Chemicals) is dissolved in Dichloromethane to make an Iodogen solution and evaporated to dryness at 20°C in sterile propylene tubes. The Iodogen reagent thus coats the inside of these tubes which are used for the labelling procedure. To this tube 10 mCi (400 MBq) ^{123}I, 0.1-0.2 ml 0.1M citrate buffer pH6, 400 ug HMFG2 (2 mg/ml in 0.1M citrate/Trist buffer pH 7.4) and 10 ul Potassium Iodide (6 x 10^{-5}M in water) are added and mixed together by gentle shaking for 10 minutes. To remove free ^{123}I the mixture is decanted onto a Sephadex G50 filtration column in a 20 ml syringe which has been pre-washed with 1% serum albumin in phosphate buffered saline. After a 5 ml void volume, the eluate is collected, activity assayed and passed through a micropore filter into sterile vials. Chromatographic quality control is undertaken and the reagent used if there has been over 70% labelling efficiency. Using the iodogen technique in this way, the immunoreactivity and avidity of a monoclonal antibody of class IgG_1 such as anti-human milk fat globule antigen, HMFG2 or anti-neuro-blastoma cell line UJI3A, as determined by direct immunoassay is unaltered.

Technique of imaging with ^{123}I labelled monoclonal antibody

The patient is selected as appropriate by the surgeon or medical oncologist. The nature of the test is explained to the patient and informed signed consent is obtained. Potassium iodide 60 mg is given orally the day before, during and for three days after the test. In addition Potassium Perchlorate 400 mg may be given just before the injection. An intradermal skin test with 0.1 ml of the antibody is performed at least 30 min. before the test and compared with a control injection of saline to check for any sensitivity to mouse protein.

Provided the skin test is negative, the patient is then positioned supine on the scanning couch. The gamma camera, e.g. Siemens large field of view ZLC 37 tube, fitted with a high resolution, low energy, parallel hole collimator and peaked for ^{123}I with a 20% window, is placed anteriorly over the pelvis. The injection of 3-4 mCi (120-160 MBq) of ^{123}I HMFG2 containing less than 0.4 mg of monoclonal antibody is given intravenously into the right antecubital vein. Dynamic studies are recorded at a 30 s framing rate for the first 4.5 min. directly into e.g. a DEC gamma 11 computer. Static images are then taken at 10 minutes, at 4 hours and at 22 hours. anteriorly and posteriorly over the lower chest, abdomen and pelvis together with separate marker scans. For the latter the patient's bony landmarks, xiphisternum, costal margins, anterior superior iliac spines, and symphysis pubis are marked with indelible ink and point source radioactive markers are positioned over these. Transparent films of the marker positions on the persistence scope are made at the early visit. At each subsequent visit, the markers are repositioned on the patient and the patient is repositioned until the image of the marker on the persistence scope fits that on the previously recorded film positioned over the scope. The computer is also programmed so that the recorded images can be moved and fixed one pixel at a time, vertically, horizontally or by rotation so that an exact superimposition of the later image over the earlier image may be made in order that detailed analysis of the images may be performed using proportional subtraction techniques or temporal change detection algorithms which produce probability maps of the sites of significant uptake. In our experience images later than 22 hours have not been required.

Tissue Background Correction

In order to make use of a high activity short lived radionuclide attached to an antibody which has low uptake by the tissue or tumour of interest, it is necessary to make some correction for the activity in the non tumour environment and blood background. This was first approached by using an agent confined to the blood pool such as $^{99}Tc^m$ albumin or extracellular fluid such as $^{99}Tc^m$ DTPA. The distributions of these agents were subtracted from the antibody distribution. However there are major theoretical and practical problems due to the different gamma ray energy of the background agent $^{99}Tc^m$ and the antibody label ^{131}I as reviewed by Ott et al[5]. A physical approach to the reduction of dual radionuclide image subtraction artefacts in immunoscintigraphy is described by Perkins et al [6] and the most successful way of overcoming this problem is undertaken by Green et al[7].

The approach that has been used in this department is to use the distribution of ^{123}I labelled antibody early after injection at a time, 10 mins, when the blood pool effect is large and the tumour uptake is small as the reference image with which images taken at later times, 4 hr. and 22 hr. are compared. Initially the tumour image enhancement was undertaken by subtracting progressive fractions of the early image from the later image in order to identify the sites of abnormal uptake[8]. More recently change detection algorithms have been applied. This approach is based on the evidence that tumour uptake increases with time, probablly following Michaelis Menten kinetics whereas tissue background and blood pool activity falls with time. By looking at the series of images 10 min, 4 hr., 22 hr., pixel by pixel, the direction of change of activity can be detected and analysed. The probability that such a change is significant can be tested and the distribution of the sites of high probability of positive and negative change can be mapped. Thus a new display of the data is derived so that highly significant increases with time, $P<0.001$, may for example be portrayed in red, $P<0.05$ in orange, and $P<0.01$ in yellow. This approach has enabled the detection of biopsy proven viable tumour sites 0.5 cm across in the peritoneum[9]. These techniques require high count rates as obtained using ^{123}I and careful superimposition of the images taken at each time. Therefore a patient repositioning protocol as described above is followed by an image repositioning protocol in the computer: First the radioactive marker images are analysed to find the pixels of highest count content so that superimposition of the patient marker images is accurate through algorithms enabling one image to be moved one pixel at a time in any direction [10]. The patient's images are then superimposed in the same way and tested for accuracy of superimposition with respect to obvious features such as activity in blood vessels. After superimposition, the change detection algorithms are applied[11].

Clinical Studies

The opportunity presented itself to study a child with neuroblastoma on two occcasions, the first with ^{131}I labelled UJ13A and the second with ^{123}I labelled UJ13A four months later to recalculate the therapeutic ratio of tumour to liver to see if therapy with the radioiodinated antibody would be beneficial. In each study the child received 1 mCi (40 MBq) of radioiodinated antibody. With ^{131}I UJI3A the tumour could not be seen until 72 hours and then only as diffuse uptake with poor resolution, whereas with ^{123}I UJ13A the tumour was clearly localised as a focal area of increased uptake at 22 hours separate from the spleen. This is reported in detail elsewhere[12]. This case illustrates the importance of the high count rate from a short lived radionuclide with good statistical information in improved detectability over the same administered dose of a long lived low count radionuclide, even although the apparent signal to noise ratio is potentially better at 72 hours than at 22 hours due to the greater tissue and background clearance of the unattached labelled antibody at that time.

The assessment of radiolabelled monoclonal antibody imaging of cancer has been largely comparative, where the interpretation of the images has been undertaken in the knowledge of whether the patient had cancer or not, of whether metastases were likely to be present or not and even of whether the radiological findings were abnormal. This is the legitimate part of the learning process in the development of a new imaging technique. It helps to establish a feel for the normal and abnormal appearances but does not help to assess the clinical efficacy of the test. After demonstrating the good imaging capabilities of ^{123}I HMFG2 in ovarian and colon cancer, a prospective study was undertaken which will be reported in detail elsewhere[9,13]. The next 30 patients referred by the gynaecologist or medical oncologist were studied in the nuclear medicine department consecutively in the absence of clinical data. Independently made maps of the distribution of uptake of the antibody were compared with maps of the surgical findings also made independently. The conclusions were that using the labelled antibody as a screening test for ovarian cancer in patients presenting with a pelvic mass of unknown aetiology was unsuccessful. This was because of the lack of specificity of the antibody with uptake in metastases from the stomach and colon carcinoma and hepatoma as well as uptake in large benign ovarian tumour. However in patients with ovarian cancer the correlation of the antibody maps and the surgical drawings were very good both before the primary operation and after full chemotherapy before the second look operation. These findings indicate that the major use of radio-immuno-scintigraphy will be in defined clinical circumstances such as, for example, the assessment of the effects of chemotherapy in order to reduce the need for a 'second look' operation, or in the demonstration of uptake in metastases as a prelude to intraperitoneal therapy.

Conclusion

The improvements in radioimmunoscintigraphy will come by recognising the superiority of ^{123}I and ^{111}In over ^{131}I as the label; by improving the uptake of the radiopharmaceutical through the use of monoclonal antibodies of higher avidity and better specificity; and by more sophisticated analysis of the sequential imaging data through change detection algorithms.

Table I   RADIONUCLIDES FOR LABELLING ANTIBODIES
          IMAGING

	123_I	111_{In}	131_I	$99_{Tc}m$
Half life	13 h	67 h	8 days	6 h
Gamma ray energy Kev	159	171 250	364	140
Beta particle energy Kev	none	none	610	none
Suitability for gamma camera				
Crystal absorption	excellent	very good	poor	excellent
Thin collimator	yes	no	no	yes
Ease of labelling	good	moderate	very good	poor
Availability	weekly	twice weekly	daily	twice daily
Injected dose, m Ci	3-4	3-4	1-2	10+
Radionuclide cost per injected dose	75	200	25	10

REFERENCES

1. Wahl, R.L., Parker C.W. Philpott G.
   Improved radioimaging and tumour localisation with monoclonal
   F(ab')$_2$.
   J. Nucl. Med. 1983; 24: 316-325.

2 Begent R.H.J., Keep P.A., Green A.J. Searle F. Bagshawe K.D.
   Jewkes R.F., Jones B.E., Barratt G.M., Ryman B.E.
   Liposomally entrapped second antibody improves tumour
   imaging with radio labelled (first)anti-tumour antibody.
   Lancet 1983; ii:739-741.

3. Park C.H., Ebbert M.A., Murphy P.R.
   Factors influencing DTPA conjugation with antibodies by
   cyclic DTPA anhydride.
   J. Nucl. Med. 1983; 24:1158-1163.

4. Fairweather D.S., Bradwell A.R., Dykes P.W., Vaughan A.T.,
   Watson-James S.F., Chandler S.
   Improved tumour localisation using Indium-111 labelled
   antibodies.
   Brit. med. J. 1983; 287: 167-170.

5. Ott R.J., Grey L.J., Zivanovic M.A., Flower M.A.,
   Trott N.G., Moshakis V., Coombes R.C., Neville A.M.,
   Ormerod M.G., Westwood J.H.
   Limitations of dual radionuclide subtraction technique for
   detection of tumours by radio-iodine labelled antibodies.
   Brit. J. Radiol. 1983; 56: 101-108.

6. Perkins A.C., Whalley D.R., Hardy J.G.
   Physical approach for the reduction of dual radionuclide
   immage subtraction artefacts in immunoscintigraphy.
   Nucl. Med. Commun. 1984; 5: 510-512.

7. Green A.J., Begent R.H.J., Keep P.A., Bagshawe K.E.
Analysis of radioimmunodetection of tumours by the
subtraction technique.
J. Nucl. Med. 1984; 25: 96–100.

8. Granowska M., Britton K.E. Shepherd J.
The detection of ovarian cancer using ^{123}I monoclonal
antibody. Radiobiol. Radiother. 1984; 25: 153–160.

9. Granowska M., Shepherd J., Britton K.E., Ward B., Mather S.,
Carroll M.J., Nimmon C.C., Slevin M.
^{123}I labelled monoclonal antibody imaging in ovarian
cancer, a prospective study in comparison with the surgical
findings. Submitted for publication.

10. Carroll M.J., Flatman W.D., Nimmon C.C., Granowska M.,
Britton K.E.
Congruent image registration as a prerequisite for detailing
sequential changes during radioimmunoscintigraphy.
Nucl. Med. Commun. 1984 ; 5:230–1.

11. Nimmon C.C., Carroll M.J., Flatman W.D., Marsden P.
Granowska M., Horne T., Britton K.E.
Spatial probability mapping of temporal change: application
to gamma camera quality control and immunoscintigraphy.
Nucl. Med. Commun. 1984; 5:231.

12. Granowska M., Dicks-Mirieux C., Britton K.E., Mather S.,
Kemshead J.T., Goldman A., Gordon I.
Imaging strategy with ^{123}I and ^{131}I labelled
monoclonal antibody, an illustrative case report:
in preparation.

13. Granowska M., Shepherd J., Britton K.E., Ward B., Mather S.,
Taylor-Papadimitriou J., Epenetos A.A., Carroll M.J.,
Nimmon C.C., Hawkins L.A., Slevin M., Flatman W., Horne T.

65

Burchell J., Durbin H. & Bodmer W.
Ovarian cancer : diagnosis using ^{123}I monoclonal antibody in comparison with surgical findings.
Nucl. Med. Commun. 1984; 5: 485–499.

Specific and non specific mechanisms in the Radio-immunodetection of tumours

Oehr P. and Winkler C.

Institute of Clinical and Experimental Nuclearmedicine
University of Bonn, Bonn , FRG.

Attempts to apply antisera in the treatment of cancer date
back to the second half of the last century (6,13). This has lead to
the idea that it might be possible to produce radioactive labelled
antibodies for tumour localization.   Pioneer achievements in this
field go back to work by Pressman and Bale et al. (22,23,1). These
authors were successful in separating gammaglobulines, which after
labelling with radioiodine and i.v injection in tumour bearing mice
or rats, accumulated selectively in malignant tissues. It was also
possible to show the fixation of the radioactive substrates in
tumour sediments in vitro.

To a certain extent, however, the assumption drawn from the
early experiments that the accumulation of radioactivity was due
to binding of antibodies to tumour-specific antigens has to be
restricted because part of the results achieved had to be
attributed to binding of gammaglobuline to fibrin present in
tumours (11, 2). Increased fibrin content is especially found in
rapidly growing malignancies both in experimental tumours and in
human malginancies. Fig. 1 shows the scintigraphic proof of fibrin
accumulation in multiple Jensen sarcomas in a rat.

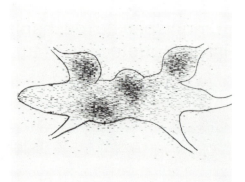

Fig 1. ^{131}J-labelled Fibrin Antibodies localized in Multiple Jensen Sarcomas

We have also been able to use increased fibrin deposition in a human osteogenic sarcoma as the basis for imaging of the tumour (Fig.2) A new immunological approach to tumour localization by means of scintigraphy is based on investigations of Bjorlund who isolated from the homogenate of a large number of varied tumours a protein-like substance which he called Tissue Polypeptide Antigen (TPA) (3,4,5). Antibodies directed against this substance revealed a cytotoxic effect on tumour cells. In work based on Bjorklund's results Gold and Freeman later isolated a further tumour constituent by extraction with perchloric acid. The substrate was called carcinoembryonic antigen (CEA) (9,10). The afore mantioned as well as other tumour associated substances i.e. alpha-fetoprotein (AFP) or human chorionic gonadotropin (HCG) have since achieved great significance as tumour markers for the follow-up in malignant diseases. However, it must be noted that the antigens are also present in normal tissues and especially in

68

inflammatory regions.

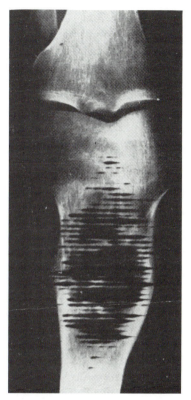

Fig.2. Radioimmunodetection of an Ostenogenic Sarcoma by means of Anti-Fibrin Antibodies (Fotoscan)

Goldenberg has recently produced polyclonal antibodies directed against CEA and has examined their potential use for radioimmunodetection (RID) (11,12). Later on Mach developed a technique using monoclonal anti-CEA antibodies in order to increase the specificity (14,15). Further development was concerned with the improvement of antibody accumulation in cancer by the use of enzymatically produced antibody fragments (15). In addition, attempts were made to apply double antibody techniques whereby first a heterologous antibody was injected and afterwards a second radioactive labelled antibody which was directed against the first one. Investigations carried out by our group together with Björklund referred specifically to the application of anti-TPA (19). We were able to show that through suitable purification procedures it was possible to produce anti-TPA antibodies which are stored and metabolized in the liver, but in smaller amounts than was the case with most of the preparations hitherto used for RID.

In principal, however, it is questionable whether in the suggested antibody binding to tumour-associated substances a tumour-specific process can really be considered. As early as 1935 Duran-Reynolds reported that non-specific accumulation of globules and other macromolecules might be observed in certain tumours (7). We were able to confirm this assertation in numerous experiments with transplantable tumours. The reasons for the non-specific uptake in tumours are variable. They may be due to the altered structure of vessels, to pinocytosis or other histological changes many of which may still be unknown. From the practical point of view it is important to establish that histochemical investigations by means of affinity-purified TPA-antibodies and subsequent PAP-dyeing have shown that a considerable uptake can also be observed in non-malignant inflammatory areas. Appropriate effects could also be achieved in vivo. Fig.3 represents radiolabelled anti-TPA accumulations in inflammatory areas caused by heat coagulation of muscle tissue in tumour-free animals. The reason for this could be an increased perfusion and/or binding of antibodies to released TPA (Fig.4,5)

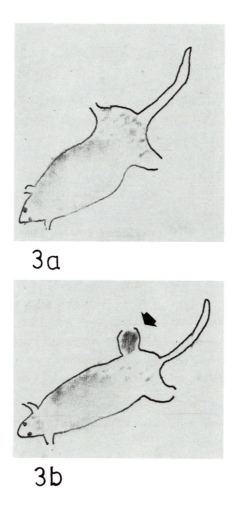

Fig.3 a–b   Radiolabelled accumulations in inflammatory area of
a rat
3 a – before inflammation
3b – inflammation caused by heat coagulation in hind leg.

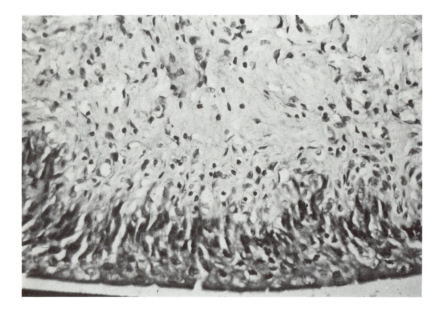

Fig. 4. Weak positive staining for TPA in animal inflammatory urothelium of the bladder.

This is supported by the fact that we were able to show increased TPA-concentration in the plasma when inflammatory processes were present Tab.1)

It is interesting to note that sarcomas are generally TPA-negative. This is agreement with the fact that up to now TPA has only been observed in epithelial tissues (18). As far as protein fragments are concerned it might be possible for these small molecules to penetrate the walls of stroma vessels and thus to accumulate in the intestine. We found significant radioactivity uptake in bladder carcinoma in ACI-rats following the injection of non specific donkey-anti-rabbit $F(ab)_2$-fragments (Fig.6).

Mechanisms of this kind as mentioned above are probably at least partly responsible for the results published by some groups in which a specific binding to tumour-antigens was assumed.

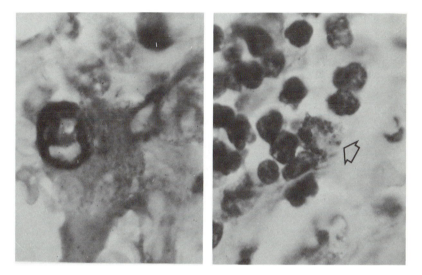

5a   5b

Fig 5. a-b Positive staining for TPA released from a necrotic cell.   5 a – necrotic cell releasing TPA
    5 b – released TPA

In order to be able to assess the relevance of many results published to date it is also important to consider the animal model used. It is possible that antibodies directed against the tumour-associated substance of a human tumour have non-specific affinity to a transplanted tumour tissue. We discovered for example by means of immune histological dyeing that unspecific horse antibodies (IgG-fraction) were preferentially bound to

73

Walker- carcinosarcomas but not to normal body tissues such as muscle.

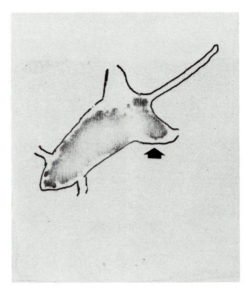

Fig. 6. Uptake of radioactivity in a bladder carcinoma transplanted into the hind leg of a rat following the injection of non specific donkey anti-rabbit $F(ab)_2$-fragments.

This phenomenon must also be taken into account when, for example, the accumulation of anti-CEA in human tumours growing in nude mice is established. As already mentioned it has also yet to be clarified to what extent increased perfusion of tumour tissues or in general the chaotic environment characterised by inflammatory changes are important in the localization of immune proteins (2).

In order to avoid problems of non-specificity, for example uptake in inflammatory areas, we proposed in 1956 a different way for the localization of antibodies in cancer (24,26). Our considerations were based in investigations by Parker, Malmgren and Mose (16,17,21) who had shown that after i.v. injection of spores of anaerobic bacteria germination occurs exclusively in the anaerobic milieu of malignant tumours. Fig.7 shows the gram- dyed bacteria of Clostridium butyricum growing in the intestice of a Yoshida Sarcoma.

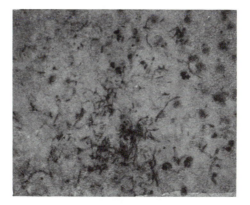

Fig. 7. Bacteria of Cl. butyricum germinated in a Yoshida Sarcoma.

We were able to show that antibodies raised against these apathogenic bacteria accumulated selectively in Walker carcinomas, Jensens sarcomas and Yoshida-sarcomas when the animals has previously been injected with clostridia spores. In recent years this technique has been further developed especially with regard to the production of highly purified antibodies directed against specific epitopes of the bacteria used. Through the application of double-antibody technique (ab 1 = anti-clostridia-ab produced in rabbits, as 2 = anti-rabbit-ab labelled by radioiodine) it might be possible to increase the amount of accumulated radioactivity in the tumour tissue. In addition experimental investigations are currently being performed in order to check as to what extent F (ab)$_2$-fragments of the immune proteins result in further optimization of RID.

One of the most recent approaches to antibody localization in malignomas is the use of antibodies raised against antigens expressed on the cell surface of specific tumours. The development of methods of cloning antibody-producing cells has led to the idea of the application of highly specific anti-tumour antibodies for RID. However, this possibility seems also to be still in an experimental stage.

It has been generally stated that improved knowledge of the exact localization of the antibodies in the tumour tissue would seem to be of decisive importance for the further development of RID. Autoradiography and immunofluorescence are particularly suitable for investigations of this kind. We have used both methods in connection with the application of anti-TPA antibodies and of anti-clostridia antibodies. The use of a new generation of fluorochrome (Biofluan) has proved to be extremely helpful, the reason for this being the absence of fading-effects which are normally found in fluorescence-dyes. The fluorescent dye synthetised by us was couple to histamine groups of immune proteins (20). In the course of immuno-histological investigations we were able to establish that the new procedure has significant advantages in comparison with the use of fluorochrome like fluoresce-inoisotiocyanate or texas red. The microphotographical documentation of the binding sites can be optimally achieved and has already led to more far reaching discoveries than hitherto possible. An example of the immuno- histological demonstration of the localization of anti-TPA antibodies in epithelial tissue is shown in fig.8 where the cytoskeleton appears clearly differentiated. The application of Biofluan-labelled TPA antibodies could perhaps also be of use for the microscopic detection of tumour tissue during a surgical operation in order to control the complications of the tumour removal.

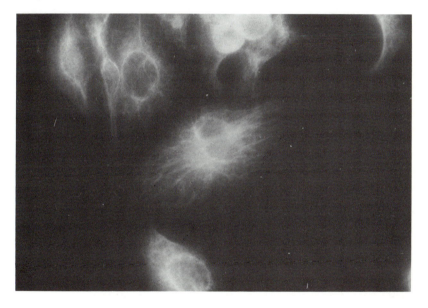

Fig.8 Staining of TPA in interphase HeLa cells by indirect immunofluorescence

Table 1.

Location	No. of Samples	elevated(%)
lung	25	29
intestine	27	18
urinary bladder	50	38

Tab. 1 Increased TPA–concentrations in plasma of patients with imflammatory processes. Cut–off level for TPA–concentration at 95% specificity of healthy persons.

REFERENCES

1. Bale, W.F., Spar, I.L. Goodland, R.L., Wolfe, D.E.: In Vivo and in Vitro Studies of labelled Antibodies Against Rat Kidney and Walker Carcinoma. Proc. Soc. Exp. Biol. Med. 89, 564–568, 1955.

2. Bale, W.F., Contreras, M.A., and Grady, E.D.: Factors Influencing Localization of Labelled Antibodies in Tumors. Cancer Res. 40, 2965–2972, 1980.

3. Bjorklund, B.: Antigenicity of Malignant and Normal Human Tissues by Gel Diffusion Techniques. Int. Arch. Allergy 8,179, 1956.

4. Bjorklund, B., Graham, J.B., and Graham, R.M.: Effect of horse Anti-Human Cancer Serum on Malignant and Normal Human Cells. Int. Arch. Allergy 10, 56, 1957.

5. Bjorklund, B., and Bjorklund, V.: Antigenicity of Pooled Human Malignant and Normal Tissues by Cyto–Immunological Technique: Frequence of an Insoluble, Heat-Labile Tumor Antigen. Int. Arch. Allergy 10, 153, 1957.

6. Busch, E.: Verh. Niederrhein. Ges. f. Natur- u. Heilkunde zu

Bonn. Berl. Klin. Wschr. 3, 1966.

7. Duran-Reynolds, F., Studies on the Localization of Dye and Foreign Proteins in Normal and Malignant Tissues. Am. J. Cancer 35, 1939.

8. Ghose, T., Tai, J., Guclu, A., Norwell, S.T., Bodurtha, A., Aquino, J., and McDonald, A.S.: Antibodies as Carriers of Radionuclides and Cytotoxic Drugs in the Treatment and Diagnosis of Cancer, An.. N.Y. Acad. Sci. 277, 671–689, 1976.

9. Gold, P., and Freedman, S.O.: Specific Carcinoembryonic Antigens of the Human Digestive System. J. Exp. Med. 122, 467, 1965.

10. Gold, P., and Freedman, S.O.: Tests for Carcinoembryonic Antigen. Role in Diagnosis and Management of Cancer. J. Am. Med. Ass. 234, 190, 1975.

11. Goldenberg, D., Preston, D.F. Primus F.J.: Photoscan Localization of GW–39 Tumors in Hamsters Using Radiolabelled Anticarcinoembryonic Antigen Immunoglobulin G. Cancer Res. 34, 1–9, 1974.

12. Goldenberg, D.M., Kim, E.E. Deland, F., Spremulli, E., Nelson M.O. Lockerman, J.P., Primus F.J., Corgan, R.L., and Alpert, E.: Clinical Studies on the Radioimmunodetection of Tumors Containing Alpha–Fetoprotein. Cancer (Phila.). 45, 2500–2505, 1980.

13. Hericourt, J., and Richet, C.: Traitement d'un Case de Sarcome par la Serotherapie. C.R. Hebd. Seances Acad. Sci. 120, 948–950, 1895.

14. Mach. J.P., Forni, M., Ritschard, J., Buchegger, F., Carrel, S., Widgren, S., Donath, A., Alberto, P.: Use and Limitations of Radiolabelled Anti-CEA Antibodies for Photoscanning Detection of Human Colorectal Carcinomas. Oncodevelopmental Biology and

D

Medicine, 1, 49–69, 1980. Biomedical Press Elsevier/North–Holland.

15. Mach, J.P., Buchegger F., Haskell, C., Schreyer, M., Carrel, S.: Selection of New Monoclonal Antibodies Against CEA and their Fragments for Detection of Carcinomas by Immunoscintigraphy. Presentation at the XI Annual Meeting of the International Society for Oncodevelopmental Biology and Medine, Stockholm, Sweden, Sept. 11–15, 1983, Abstract P.93.

16. Malmgreen, R.A., Flanigan, C.C.: Localisation of the Vegetative Form of Clostridium Tetani in Mouse Tumours Following Intravenous Spore Administration. Cancer Res. 15, 1955.

17. Mose, J.R., and Mose, G.: Onkolyseversuch mit apathogenen, anaeroben Sporenbildern am Ehrlich–Tumor der Maus. Z. Krebsforschung 63. 1959.

18. Nathrath, W.B.J., Heidenkummer, P., Arnholdt, H., Bassermann R., Lohrs, U., Permanetter, W., Remberger, K., and Wiebecke B: Distrubtion of Tissue Polypeptide Antigen (TPA) in Normal and Neoplastic Human Tissues. XXXIst Colloquium, Protides of the Biological Fluids, Ed. H. Peeters, Pergamon Press, 1984, in press.

19. Oehr, P., Björklund, B., Biersack, H.J., and Winkler, C.: Radioimmunodetection by Anti-TPA-Antibodies. Int. Ass. Radiopharmcol., Third Intern. Symp. on Radiopharmacol., Freiburg, Sept. 21–25, 1983, Abstract, P.57.

20. Oehr, P., Winkler, C., Reichel, C., Watzek, C.,: A New Generation of Dyes for Fluerimetric Detection of Protides in Biological Fluids. Proc. XXXII. Colluqu. Protides of the Biological Fluids, Abstract, 1984.

21. Parker, R.C., Plummer, H.C., Siebenmann, C.O., Chapmann, M.G.: Effect of Histolyticus Infections and Toxins on Transplantable Mouse Tumors. Proc. Soc. Exper. Biol. Med. 66,

1947.

22. Pressman, D.: The Zone of Activity of Antibodies as Determined by the Use of Radioactive Tracers. Ann. N.Y. Acad. Sci. 11, 203–206, 1949.

23. Pressman, D., and Pressman, R.,: Computer Programs for Paired and Triad Radioiodine Label Techniques in Radioimmunochemistry. Int. J. Appl. Radiat. Isotop. 18, 617, 622, 1965.

24. Schubert, R., Winkler, C.: Selektive Radioaktivitatsanreicherungen in Tumoren. Untersuchungen ueber die Moglichkeit der Fixation markierter Antikorper an intratumoral wachsende Bakterien. Fortschritte d. Medzin 83/9, 1965.

25. Spar, I.L., Goodland, R.L., Bale, W.F.: Localization of ^{131}J-Labelled Antibody to Rat Fibrin in a Transplantable Rat Lymphosarcoma. Proc. Soc. Exp. Biol. Med. 100, 259–262, 1959.

26. Winkler, C.: Uber die Nutzung gerinnungsphysiologischer und immunologischer Prozesse fur die Radioaktivitatsanreicherung in Tumoren. In: Radioisotope in der klinischen und experimentellen Onkologie, Schattauer-Verlag Stuttgart, 1965, P.349.

Kinetic Distribution studies *in Vivo* of Radioiodinated Monoclonal preparations as a screening procedure for tumour immunoscintigraphy agents.

Mariani G., Mazzucca N., Molea N., Bianchi R. and Donato L.

CNR Institute of Clinical Physiology; 5th Medical Pathology and Nuclear Medicine Service of the University of Pisa; PISA (Italy).

INTRODUCTION

The identification of specific tumour-associated antigens has provided the experimental basis for developing techniques for the in vivo detection of tumour lesions by means of external radioimmunoscintigraphy. Such techniques were preliminarily applied using labelled antibodies obtained from conventional, polyclonal antisera raised against CEA (1,2), alpha-fetoprotein (3), HCG (4), ferritin (5), and a kidney cercinoma antigen (6). However, low titre and heterogeneity of polyclonal antisera limit the clinical validity of the results obtained, due to the cross-reactivity with tissues and organs in the body, and to the relatively low localization of the labelled antibodies in the tumour as compared with the fraction remaining in circulating blood or to the nonspecific accumulation in the liver and spleen.

Monoclonal antibodies represent a distinct breakthrough in this respect, due to their advantageous properties with respect to high titre and specificity. Since the first production of monoclonal antibodies by Kohler and Milstein (7), immunological tools in general have in fact gained a renewed impetus for incisive investigations in various areas, including experimental and clinical oncology (8).

Investigations on the in vivo distribution of labelled anti-tumour monoclonal preparations were undertaken in this study, with the purpose of evaluating to what extent the kinetics of plasma disappearance combined with the kinetics of both nonspecific tissue uptake and specific uptake at tumour sites may affect the quality of scintigraphic images obtained at subsequent times after injection of a particular monoclonal tracer.

MATERIALS AND METHODS

Monoclonal Tracers

Three types of monoclonal preparation were studied. Hybridoma 225.28S produced anti-human melanoma IgG_{2a} immunoglobulins that have been successfully used to radioimage human melanoma lesions both in the nude-mouse model (9) and in melanoma patients (10). Anti-CEA monoclonal IgG_1 immunoglobulins were produced by hybridoma F023C5 (11), while hybridoma 16B13 produced IgG_{2a} antibodies against human lung cancer (including oat cell carcinoma) (12).

Both labelled intact IgGs and labelled F(ab')2 fragments were studied in the case of clones 225.28S and F023C5, while in the case of clone 16B13 only the kinetics of F8ab')2 was determined. Details on production of the antibodies, their purification, preparation of the F(ab')2 fragments, labelling with I-131 and testing of the specific in vitro immunoreactivity after radiolabelling are reported elsewhere in this volume by Callegaro and coworkers (13). 225.28S tracer was studied at two distinct specific activity ranges (1.5–3.5 mCi/mg and 45–55 mCi/mg respectively), while FO23C5 and 16B13 tracers had specific activities in the 8–16 mCi/mg range.

Patients

Hospitalized cancer patients only were included in this study, after informed consent had been obtained. Before intravenous administration of the monoclonal tracers, patients were tested for hypersensitivity to mouse immunoglobulins by injecting 3.0–3.5 ug mouse IgG intradermally. Thyroidal radioiodine uptake was blocked by potassium iodide (120 mg daily for 10 days, starting 3 days prior to tracer injection).

A total of 26 patients were studied, of whom 13 patients received the anti–melanoma preparations (:^{131}I-225.28S–IgC$_{2a}$ in 8 cases, and ^{131}I-225.28S–F(ab')2 in 5 cases), 8 patients received the anti–CEA tracers (^{131}I-F023C5–IgG$_1$ and ^{131}I-F023C5–F(ab')2 in 4 cases each), and 5 patients were injected with the ^{131}I-16B13–F(ab')2 anti–lung cancer tracer. The patients were affected by tumours different from those for which the injected tracers were expected to be specific, except for two patients in the 16B13 tracer group, who were in fact affected by lung cancer (an oat cell and a squamous cell carcinoma, respectively).

Protocol for the Distribution Studies

The radiotracer solution (2 to 5 ml, containing 0.5 to 1 mCi) was injected i.v. over a 1–minute period. Heparinized venous blood samples were taken 5 minutes after completing injection, then at adequately timed intervals until 6 days thereafter, to determine the plasma disappearance curves of the injected tracers. A whole

-body LFOV gamma camera (73 photomultipliers, KR7 SELO, Milan, Italy) connected on-line with a dedicated computer (Medusa ULP/12, SEPA, Turin, Italy) was used for the scintigraphic recording, using a medium-energy, parallel-hole collimator (setting at 364 keV, with a 30% window). Whole-body scans were recorded shortly after injection (within one hour), then at daily intervals until 6 days after injection, with the patients always in the same geometrical conditions. All the scintigraphic images were recorded using a 128x128 matrix. Specific regions of interest (ROIs) for the relevant organs (routinely liver and spleen, but also other organs when adequate) were defined over the displayed images and the relative radioactivity concentrations were determined.

Data Analysis

Analysis of the in vivo and in vitro data obtained allowed to derive sets of parameters concerning the kinetics of tracer disappearance from circulating plasma, the overall retention of radioactivity in the body at subsequent times after tracer injection and the kinetics of activity distribution to the liver and spleen (or other organs when investigated). The plasma disappearance curves of the monoclonal tracers were analyzed according to the integral or noncompartmental approach (14), using classical formulae to compute the mean transit time (t) and the total metabolic clearance rate (MCR) of the tracers, considered as the overall sum of clearing mechanisms operating in the body upon tracer injection. These include both degradation of the protein preparations through catabolic processes occurring within or in spaces exchanging rapidly with the plasma space, and tracer accumulation in various organs and tissues, such as the liver, spleen, and bone marrow.

RESULTS

Overall Scintigraphic results

The anti-tumour monoclonal tracers never showed any uptake at known tumour sites in patients affected by tumours different from those for which the antibodies were expected to be specific.

A markedly different pattern of distribution was observed for the two anti-melanoma tracers derived from clone 225.28S. ^{131}I-225.28S-IgG$_{2a}$ rapidly accumulated at a high extent in the liver, spleen and bone marrow; resulting scintigraphic images were therefore similar to thos obtained after administration of a typical bone marrow imaging radiopharmaceutical, as shown in Figure 1A. This feature was not observed with ^{131}I-225.28S-F(ab')2, which exhibited a scintigraphic pattern similar to those observed with both IgG and F(ab')2 tracers from anti-CEA clone F023C5, characterized by some nonspecific uptake in the liver and spleen and by a more diffuse and homogeneous extravascular distribution, starting from a few hours after injection (Fig. 1B). As concerns the anti-lung cancer, ^{131}I-F(ab')2 from clone 16B13, this tracer consistently showed a significant and persistent uptake in the normal lungs, of approximately the same intensity as that observed in both liver and spleen (Fig. 2). Due to this fact, it was not possible to determine the differential tracer accumulation in specific ROIs, because of the overlap of the liver and spleen with adjacent lung regions. Conversely, ^{131}I-16B13F(ab')2 did not show any appreciable specific uptake on the known tumour sites in the two patients affected by lung cancer.

87

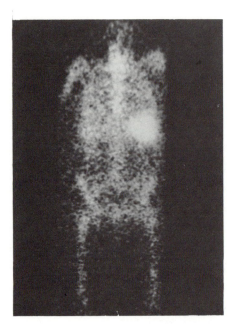

Figure 1A.

Scintigraphic image of the whole body obtained 24 hours after the injection of ^{131}I-225.28S–IgG$_{2a}$: marked uptake in the spleen, liver, and overall reticulo–endothelial system, with scintigraphic appearance as with a typical bone-morrow imaging radiopharmaceutical.

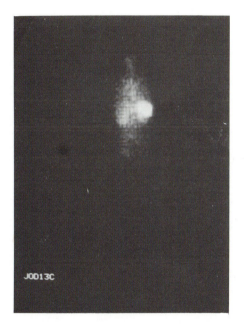

Figure 1B.

Scintigraphic image of the whole body obtained 24 hours after the injection of ^{131}I-225.28S–F(ab)$_2$: some residual significant uptake is detected in the spleen, whereas the remaining radioactivity is quite homogeneously diffused in the blood space and the extravascular spaces. Scintigraphic images of this type were also obtained after injection of ^{131}I-tracers from clone F023C5 (either whole IgG$_1$ and F(ab')$_2$), with even lower nonspecific accumulations in the liver and spleen.

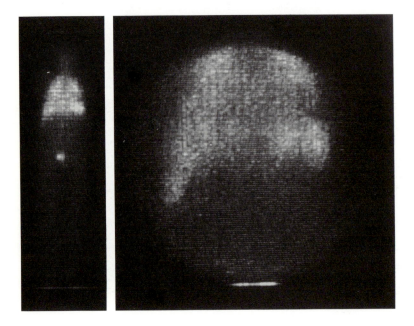

Figure 2.

Scintigraphic images of the whole body (on the left) and of the chest and upper abdomen (on the right) obtained 72 hours after injection of ^{131}I-16B13-F(ab')$_2$ into a patient not affected by lung cancer. Relevant and diffuse uptake of the tracer in both lungs (of approximately the same extent as in the liver and spleen, with

90

resulting negative silhouette of the central blood space (heart and large vessels).

Kinetic Distribution Parameters

Table 1 reports the mean values for the kinetic distribution parameters determined in each group of patients tested with that particular monoclonal tracer. A highly homogeneous kinetic pattern was observed for each preparation, with computed standard deviation values never exceeding 10 % of the corresponding means values, particularly at early times after injection (at least until 72-96 hours post-injection). On the contrary, different monoclonal tracers were often characterized by markedly different kinetic behaviour in vivo, as shown by the parameters listed in Table 1. The figures given in the Table for the percent liver and spleen uptakes relative to whole body activity are those determined from the scans recorded one hour after tracer injection, at which time uptake in these organs is already maximum. Liver and spleen activities subsequently decline with slopes that do not differ widely for the five tracers within each organ, while somewhat slower removal rates of radioactivity from the spleen with respect to the liver were observed. Furthermore while the spleen activity curves consistently showed a monoexponential decline throughout the experimental period, the liver curves exhibited instead a distinct biphasic pattern, with a slower slope becoming obvious about 96 to 120 hours after tracer injection.

Figure 3 diagrammatically represents the average whole-body retention curves and plasma disappearance curves obtained for the five monoclonal tracers tested. These curves are worth evaluation in view of the possible scintigraphic results in the case of specific tracer uptake by tumour lesions. In particular, when using a ^{131}I-labelled tracer, the pattern of the whole-body curve and of the corresponding plasma curve at 24, 48 and 72 hours (likely to be the optimal scanning times for such a label) provides an estimate of the radioactivity background due both to activity still in circulating blood and to activity nonspecifically absorbed in extravascular sites.

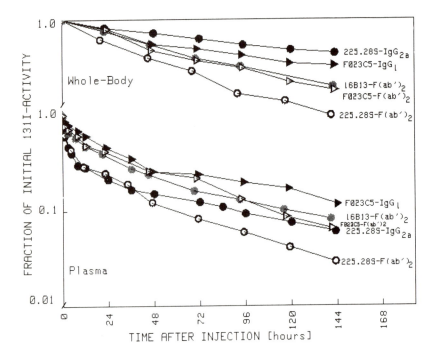

Figure 3.

Diagrammatic representation (in a semilog plot) of the whole-body surves (above) and the plasma disappearance curves (below) obtained upon injection of the five different monoclonal tracers, reported as average values for each group of observations. The relative standard deviations (not represented in the plot for the sake of clarity) never exceeded 10% of each mean value until 72–96 hours after tracer injection.

DISCUSSION

The results obtained in this work constitute a preliminary screening study for evaluating the in vivo distribution of different monoclonal preparations with potential properties as tumour radioimmunoscintigraphy agents, while providing interesting clues for the interpretation of kinetic data on the tissue distribution in vivo of monoclonal preparations from different sources.

As concerns the 225.28S preparations (anti-melanoma), data obtained with the whole IgG and with the Fab tracers showed dramatically different patterns in their tissue distribution. In fact, whole IgGs were characterized by a particularly high non-specific uptake in the reticulo-endothelial system (RES), resulting in scintigraphic images, where the high background activity would make very difficult to detect specific accumulation areas due to melanoma lesions. Furthermore, retention of the IgG tracer at the non-specific sequestration sites were very long, therefore resulting in high values of the whole-body retained activity at late times after injection (i.e., about 40% of the injected dose at 6 days). Instead, non-specific uptake in the RES was much lower for the 225.28S-F(ab')2 tracer, with resulting scintigraphic images of better quality than with 225.28S-IgG$_{2a}$. Furthermore, at different times after injection, activity in the circulation due to ^{131}I-225.28S-F(ab')2 was much lower than that due to ^{131}-225.28S-IgG$_{2a}$; this is a further advantageous feature in tumour immunoscintigraphy, since it reduces the need for dual isotope blood pool subtraction procedures. As a result of the higher removal rate, the whole-body retained activity at various

93

times following injection of ^{131}I-225.28S-F(ab')2 was much lower than after injection of ^{131}I-225.28SIgG$_{2A}$ (Fig. 3). All these findings provide the experimental evidence for the superior immunoscintigraphy properties of 225.28S-F(ab')2 with respect to intact IgG$_{2a}$ in patients with melanoma lesions, as recently reported in a parallel study (10).

The results obtained with the F023C5 preparations (anti-CEA) showed that radioiodinated whole IgG and F(ab)2 from this clone were characterized by similar patterns of early tissue distribution in vivo (at least until 48 hours after injection), with slightly lower nonspecific uptakes in the liver and spleen for ^{131}I-F023C5-Fab as compared to ^{131}I-F023C5-IgG$_1$; nonspecific sequestration in the RES was anyway moderate for both types of tracers, being considerably lower than that observed with intact IgG$_{2A}$ from clone 225.28S. General advantages in the use of F023C5-F(ab')2 versus F023C5-IgG$_1$ derive from lower circulating activities at corresponding times after injection, lower nonspecific uptakes, and lower whole-body retained activities. In keeping with these facts, a parallel study in patients with gastrointestinal cancers demonstrated the excellent radioimaging properties of F023C5-F(ab')2 tracer, whether labelled with ^{131}I or with ^{111}In (11).

The results obtained with ^{131}I-16B13-Fab (anti-human lung cancer) showed that this tracer had an overall kinetics of distribution characterized by parameters that were in some way intermediate between those of ^{131}I-IgG and ^{131}I-F(ab')2 from clone F023C5 as concerns removal constants and whole-body retained activities at various times after tracer injection. Important negative features observed for the in vivo distribution of ^{131}I-16B13-F(ab7))2 include the relevant uptake in normal lung structures and the absence of specific uptake in the lung cancer lesions studied so far. These features preclude clone 16B13 preparations from any further lung cancer immunoscintigraphy testing in vivo.

CONCLUSIONS

The overall results obtained in this study are in keeping with current reports by our group and others (10,15,16,17) in indicating the superior properties of F(ab')2 fragments with respect to intact IgG for in vivo tumour radioimmunoscintigraphy. This conclusion was obvious in the case of clone 225.28S, where the differences in the distribution patterns of IgG and Fab were particularly important, but was also pointed out in the case of clone F023C5.

As concerns the usefulness of tissue distribution studies in patients not affected by the specific tumours against which the monoclonal antibodies were raised, the results obtained in this work emphasize that the patterns of distribution and of immunoreactivity in vivo are often totally unpredictable on the basis of in vitro parameters, such as those derived from immunostaining studies on tissue sections or even from immunobinding assays with intact tumour cells in vitro. As far as in particular, the kinetics of tissue distribution is concerned, data reported in Table 1 demonstrate the large differences in the distribution parameters among different immunoglobulin classes or between intact IgG and F(ab')2 from the same clone. Furthermore, the modifications induced in the pattern of tracer distribution when changing from intact IgG to F(ab')2 from the same clone appear to be peculiar for each clone, particularly as concerns the relative proportion of nonspecific uptakes in the liver and spleen, and the corresponding removal rates from these sequestration

TABLE I - Main tissue distribution and kinetic parameters obtained for the five types of monoclonal preparations tested, reported as average values for each group.

	Kinetics of Plasma Curves			WB Activity at 144 hours % Dose	Liver Uptake % Dose	$T_{1/2}$ Liver Activity hours	Spleen Uptake % Dose	$T_{1/2}$ Spleen Activity hours
	$\bar{t}$ hours	MCR L/day	$T_{1/2}$ hours					
225.28S-IgG$_{2a}$	77.23	2.492	115.3	40	15.0	36.5	5.0	39.0
225.28S-F(ab')$_2$	53.16	4.892	36.4	10	4.5	43.0	7.5	41.0
FO23C5-IgG$_1$	101.64	1.328	85.3	28	8.7	46.1	3.0	70.6
FO23C5-F(ab')$_2$	63.35	1.917	55.3	18	7.8	37.8	2.2	55.8
16B13-F(ab')$_2$	80.72	1.965	60.2	20	(*)	38.0	(*)	50.0

$\bar{t}$ = Mean Transit Time; MCR: Total Metabolic Clearance Rate; WB = Whole-Body; $T_{1/2}$ = terminal slope.
(*) = not determined because of overlap with adjacent lung bases, showing relevant uptake of the injected tracer.

sites. Analysis of data in Table 1 also points out the differential behaviours of the reticulo-endothelial function in the liver and, respectively, in the spleen, as regards efficiency of clearing mechanism from circulating blood and subsequent local degradation rates of the uptaken tracers.

Moreover, the results obtained raise a further point, besides showing the usefulness of these studies for evaluating the tissue distribution kinetics of the individual monoclonal preparations for which a use as tumour radioimmunoscintigraphy agents is prospected. This point deals with the concept of "irrelevant monoclonal preparations" that is currently being discussed as the possible solution to the problem of differential nonspecific tissue distribution in the course of tumour immunoscintigraphy; this concept refers to the injection of an antibody tracer not directed against a tumour-associated antigen simultaneously with the specific tumour-searching tracer (17). Because of the extremely variable biological behaviour in vivo of the various monoclonal preparations, any tracer to be used for the purpose described above must preliminarily be tested, as it was done in this work, in order to ascertain that its tissue distribution kinetics is actually identical to, or at least compatible with that of the specific monoclonal tracer. On the other hand, the observed reproducibility of the distribution kinetics of each preparation in different subjects suggests that knowledge of the preparation kinetics from independent studies may be used to interpret and perhaps correct the distribution results in diagnostic studies.

REFERENCES

1. Goldenberg D.M., DeLand F., Kim E., Bennette S., Primus F.J., van Negell Jr. J.R., Estes N., DeSimone P., Rayburn P. Use of

radiolabelled antibodies to carcinoembryonic antigen for the detection and localization of diverse cancers by external photoscanning. N. Engl. J. Med., 298: 1384–1386, 1978.

2. Goldenberg D.M., Primus F.J., DeLand F. Tumour detection and localization with purified antibodies to carcinoembryonic antigen. In: Immunodiagnosis of Cancer, Vol. I, R.B. Herberman and K.R. McIntire (eds), New York, Marcel Dekker (1979), pp. 265–304.

3. Goldenberg D.M., Kim E.E., DeLand F.B., Spremulli E., Nelson M.O., Gockerman J.P., Primus F.J., Corgan R.L., Alpert E. Clinical studies on the radioimmunodetection of tumours containing alpha–fetoprotein. Cancer, 45: 2500–2505, 1980.

4. Goldenberg D.M., Kim E.E., DeLand F.H., van Nagell Jr. J.R., Javadpour N. Clinical radioimmunodetection of cancer with radioactive antibodies to human chorionic gonadotrophin. Science, 208: 1284–1286, 1980.

5. Order S.E., Bloomer W.B., Jones A.G., Kaplan W.B., Davis M.A., Adelstein S.J., Hellman S. Radionuclide immunoglobulin lymphangiography: a case report. Cancer, 35: 1487–1492, 1975.

6. Belitsky P., Glose T., Aquino J., Tai J., MacDonald A. Radionuclide imaging of metastases from renal cell carcinoma by ^{131}I-labelled antitumour antibody. Radiology, 126: 515–517, 1978.

7. Kohler G., Milstein C. Continuous cultures of fused cells secreting antibodies of predefined specificity. Nature, 256: 495–497, 1975.

8. Goldenberg D.M., DeLand F.H. History and status of tumour imaging with radiolabelled antibody. J. Biol. Response Modifiers, 1: 121–136, 1982.

9. Ghose T., Ferrone S., Imai K., Nowell S.T., Luner S.J., Martin R.H., Blair A.H. Imaging of human melanoma xenografts in nude mice with a radiolabelled monoclonal antibody. J. Natl.

Cancer Inst. 69: 823–826, 1982.

10. Buraggi G.L., Callegaro L., Ferrone S., Turrin A., Cascinelli N., Attili A., Bombardieri E., Mariani G., Deleide G. In vivo immunodiagnosis with radiolabelled antimelanoma monoclonal antibodies and F(ab')2 fragments. In: Nulearmedizin–Imaging of Metabolism and Organ Function, HAE Schmidt and WE Adam (eds), Stuttgart, Schattauer Verlag (1984), pp 713–717.

11. Buraggi G.L., Callegaro L., Turrin A., Gennari L., Bombardieri E., Gasparini M., Mariani G., Doci R., Regaglia E., Seregni E. Immunoscintigraphy of colo–rectal carcinoma: remarks about an ongoing clinical trials. In: Nuclear Medicine in Research and Practice, E. Vauramo, W.E. Adam and HAE Schmidt (eds), Stuttgart, Schattauer Verlag (1985) in press.

12. Mazauric T., Mitchell K.F., Letchworth G.J. III, Koprowski H., Steplewski Z. Monoclonal antibody defined human lung cell surface protein antigen. Cancer Res., 42: 150–154, 1982.

13. Callegaro L., Deleide G., Dovis M., Cecconato E., Plassio G. and Rosa U. Purification and labelling of F(ab')2 fragments and their conversion to radiopharmaceuticals. Proceedings of Saariselka Symposium 10–11 August 1984.

14. Gurpide E., Mann J. Interpretation of isotopic data obtained from blood borne compounds. J. Clin. Endocrinol. Metab., 30:707–719, 1970.

15. Wahl R.L., Parker C.W., Philpott G.W. Improved radioimaging and tumour localization with monoclonal F(ab')2. J. Nucl. Med., 24:316–325, 1983.

16. Mariani G., Callegaro L., Mazzucca N., Ferrone S., Rosa U., Bianchi R. In vivo distribution of anti–human melanoma monoclonal antibodies. In : Protides of the Biological Fluids, 31st, H. Peeters (ed), Oxford, Pergamon Press (1984), pp. 971–976.

17. Chatal J.F., Saccavini J.C., Fumoleau P., Douillard J.Y., Curtet C., Kremer M., LeMevel B., Koprowski H. Immunoscintigraphy of colon carcinoma. J. Nucl. Med., 25: 307–314, 1984.

Purification and labelling of F(AB')$_2$ Fragments from Anti-Tumour Monoclonal antibodies and their conversion to Radiopharmaceuticals.

Callegaro L., Deleide G., Dovis M., Cecconato E., Plassio G., Rose U. and Scassellati G.A.

Sorin Biomedica, Saluggia (Vercelli) Italy.

INTRODUCTION

The technique of tumour immunolocalization by means of radiolabelled antibodies initially started using tagged heteroantisera as tracer (1) (2) (3). However, the polyclonal antibodies showed a poor specificity and a low concentration of the immunoglobulin fraction specific for the tumour associated antigen (TAA). It was then necessary to develop affinity chromatography methods in order to isolate the specific IgG fraction (4); however, the cost of such a process is very high, because of the low yield and the need to immobilize on the solid matrix a highly purified form of the specific antigen.

Recently, the availability of monoclonal antibodies to tumour associated antigens having a high degree of specificity has contributed to more extensive in-vivo use of radiolabelled anti-tumour antibodies (5) (6) (7). It was soon obvious that, prior to the clinical applications, a lot of biochemical and radiochemical work has to be done on each monoclonal antibody and the results obtained on a single antibody cannot be extrapolated to another one, even of very similar features.

The primary goal of any study in this area is then to achieve a satisfactory reproducility of all the processes involved in the preparation of the reagents, i.e. MoAb production, MoAb labelling and quality control of labelled MoAb. Starting from the same MoAb, all the different lots of final radiotracers should present well defined and constant characteristics. Moreover, since injection into humans is the objective of this kind of study , all the specifications of a radiopharmaceutical have to be fulfilled, e.g. sterility, apyrogenicity and absence of toxicity.

The aim of our work has been primarily focussed on this aspect of the problem. We have tried to set up an "experimental protocol" capable to process any MoAb of well defined characteristics and to optimize the preparation of IgG and, whenever useful, of their F(ab')$_2$ fragments and the radiolabelling with different isotopes such as ^{131}I, ^{123}I, ^{111}In and ^{99m}Tc, warranting in the same time the pharmaceutical properties of the materials to be administered in-vivo.

MATERIALS AND METHODS

Monoclonal Antibodies

Different MoAbs were considered for this study:

. Moabs anti HMW-MAA (High Molecular Weight Melanoma Associated Antigen) 225.28S and 763.74T (8) (9) (10).

. Moabs anti LMW-MAA (Low Molecular Weight Melanoma Associated Antigen) 376.96S (10)

. MoAbs anti-CEA FO14B3, FO21D3, FO23C5 (11) (12)

. MoAb anti-Lung cell surface protein Antigen 16 B 13 (13)

. MoAb anti-HBsAg (Hepatitis B surface Antigen) 4C4 (to be used as a non specific control) (14)

102

All the IgG were obtained by mouse ascitic fluid using the caprilic acid procedure (15) and stored at -30°C until use, in 0.01 M phosphate buffered saline, pH 7.4.

F(ab')$_2$ fragments preparation

Bivalent fragments f(ab')$_2$ were prepared by pepsin digestion of monoclonal IgG following the general method of Nisonoff et al. (16) and adapting it to each particular MoAb (e.g. for the optimization of enzyme/EgG ratio). After proteolysis, the fragments were purified by gel giltration on Sephadex G-200 SF and by affinity chromatography on Protein A Sepharose CL6B (17). The purity of the final material was evaluated by SDS-slab gel electrophoresis (18).

Radiolabelling procedures

The intact IgG and their fragments were labelled with ^{131}I and ^{123}I by the iodogen method (19). Briefly 0.2 mg of IgG solution at a concentration of 3 mg/ml reacted with 12-13 mCi of ^{131}I in a tube containing 2 ug of Iodogen absorbed on the tube wall. Optimal contact time was determined to be 2 min. Unbound iodine was removed by ion exchange chromatography on Dowex resin column (1x8 cm).

The labelling with ^{111}In was caarried out by DTPA chelation method (20). The cyclic anhydride of diethylenetriamine pentaacetic acid (DTPA), stored in a desiccator at room temperature, was incubated overnight at 4°C with 2 mg F(ab')$_2$ fragments diluted in 0.1 M NaHCO$_3$ buffer, pH 8.3. The antibody conjugate was separated from unbound DTPA by desalting on Sephadex G-50 and the eluted F(ab')$_2$-DTPA was incubated for 1 hour with (^{111}In) indium chloride in 0.2 M sodium citrate buffer, pH 5.0. Unbound In was then separated from the antibody conjugate by gel filtration on Biogel P-6 (BioRad). The purity of $F(ab')_2$-DTPA conjugate was evaluated by High Pressure Liquid Chromatography (HPLC), using a gel permeation column (TSK G 3000 SW) equilibrated with 0.05M phosphate buffer pH 7,1, containg 0.3M NaCl and 0.05% sodium azide

To perform ^{99m}Tc-labelling, a solution of $F(ab')_2$ fragments in 0.04M tartrate buffer pH 6.5, containing stannous chloride and 0.01% HSA, was lyophilized at a concentration of 250 ug/vial. The freeze-dried $F(ab')_2$ fragments were than dissolved in 3 ml of a sterile solution of sodium pertechnetate (^{99m}Tc) eluted from a generator. After careful mixing, the solution was incubated for 15 minutes at room temperature. Free ^{99m}Tc was then separated from the labelled protein by ion exchange chromatography through a sterile and pyrogen-free column of anionic resin. The average labelling yield was around 80–85%.

Sterility and pyrogen tests

Radiolabelled antibodies and their $f(ab')_2$ fragments were tested for sterility and pyrogens, following the standard methods recommended by U.S. Pharmacopeia.

In vitro binding assay

Radiobinding assay using the melanoma cell line COLO 38 as specific target cells and a lymphoblastoid cell line Victor as negative control was performed in polyvinyl chloride microtiter plates (21). 200,000 cpm of radiotracer diluted in PBS solution containing 1% Bovine Serum Albumin were mixed with a cell suspension and incubated for 60 minutes at room temperature. After washing with PBS solution containing 0.1% BSA, the microtiter plates were dried and the radioactivity in each well was measured in a gamma counter.

Radiochemical purity controls

1. Radioelectrophoresis. 10 ul specimens were applied to cellulose acetate strip equilibrated with 0.1M phosphate buffer pH 7.1. After 30 min. at 200 V, the strips were counted in an automatic scanning device and the radioactivity of the relevant peaks was determined.

2. Gel chromatography. 200 ul of radiotracer were applied to a 25x0.8 cm column of Biogel P6 equilibrated with 0.15M NaCl. The column was then eluted with isotonic saline; 1 ml fractions were collected with an automatic fraction collector and their radioactivity was measured in a well scintillation counter. The presence of spurious radioactivity, remaining on the gel was checked by a radiochromatoscanner.

RESULTS AND DISCUSSION

As pointed out by the recent literature (22) (23), the F(ab')$_2$ fragments are usually preferred for in-vivo studies, in order to avoid the aspecific binding of IgG via Fc receptors and to allow a faster clearance of the radioactivity from the body, thus reducing the radioactive background and enhancing the imaging contrast.

However, each monoclonal antibody seems to present a different sensitivity to pepsin digestion: markedly different results are obtained (e.g. in terms of yield) even for MoAbs belonging to the same IgG subclass.

Table 1 summarizes the results we have obtained in the preparation of F(ab')$_2$ from IgGs of different kind, specific for different antigens (CEA, Melanoma and Lung Tumour Associated

TABLE 1

DATA RELATED TO PROTEOLYTIC DIGESTION OF DIFFERENT MONOCLONAL ANTIBODIES

CLONE, Code	ANTIGEN	IgG SUBCLASS	IgG/PEPSIN RATIO	pH	YIELD, [a] % OF PROTEIN
225.28S	HMW-MAA (1)	IgG_{2a}	50:1	4.5	12÷15
736.74T	HMW-MAA	IgG_1	50:1	4.2	20÷22
376.96S	LMW-MAA (2)	IgG_{2a}	50:1	4.5	15÷18
F023C5	CEA	IgG_1	20:1	4.0	20÷22
F021D3	CEA	IgG_{2a}	50:1	4.5	23÷25
F014B3	CEA	IgG_1	20:1	4.2	1÷2
16B13	LCSPA (3)	IgG_{2a}	50:1	4.5	25÷27
4C4	HBsAg	IgG_1	20:1	4.0	50÷55

(1) High Molecular Weight Melanoma Associated Antigen
(2) Low Molecular Weight Melanoma Associated Antigen
(3) Lung Cell Surface Protein Antigen

(a) The proteolysis was carried out at 37°C for 24 hours;

Antigens). The data related to the anti-HBsAG MoAb 4C4, used as negative control in the specificity studies, are also reported.

The results of Table 1 show that it is very difficult to set up a relationship between IgG subclass and pepsin digestion parameters, in the attempt to standardize a single procedure for $F(ab')_2$ production from antibodies of the same subclass. The optimization of the different parameters, such as enzyme/IgG ratio, incubation time, temperature and buffer pH, is essential for the success of the fragmentation process, but varies for each particular monoclonal antibody.

The purifification of $F(ab')_2$ fragments from MoAb 225.28S is reported in Fig.1. The process which has been optimized allows a routine preparation of 250 mg of purified $F(ab')_2$ for each run.

Since this monoclonal antibody had been chosen by previous studies (8) 810) (24) (25) as the best performing IgG for human melanoma in-vivo immunodetection, all the further standardization work has been carried out with this material, in the attempt to find out the most suitable radioactive tracer.

At first, by using Iodine 131, different labelling methods and different specific activities have been evaluated (21).

IgG and $F(ab')_2$ iodinated at a specific activity of 20 mCi/mg were less reactive with cultured melanoma cells Colo 38 when labelled by chloramine T or Bolton–Hunter method than when labelled by iodogen method.

By this last method, specific activities from 5 up to 50 mCi/mg could be reached without any significant impairement of the immunoreactivity as shown in Table 2: higher values of specific activity resulted in a sharp reduction of binding to the target cells Colo 38.

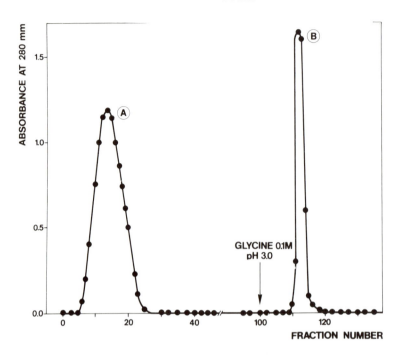

Figure 1.

Purification of F(ab')$_2$ fragments from MoAb 225.28S by affinity chromatography on Protein A-Sepharose. Fragments are eluted with void volume, while indigested IgG are eluted after equilibration of the column with 0.1 M glycine buffer pH 3.0.

This finding, which was verified also when labelling F(ab')$_2$ with ^{123}I, is probably due to the peculiar characteristics of the anti-melanoma antibody 225.28S, shown also by other studies to be an extremely robust and stable antibody. Iodinations performed later on IgGs or F(ab')$_2$ fragments from other antibodies, such as for instance the anti-CEA FO23C5, demonstrated that the maximum compatible value of specific activity ranged from 5 to 10 mCi/mg,

TABLE 2

EFFECT OF SPECIFIC ACTIVITY ON IMMUNOREACTIVITY OF RADIOIODINATED F(ab')$_2$

SPECIFIC ACTIVITY	% BINDING TO TUMOUR CELLS COLO 38
5 + 50	100 about 10.2[a]
55	88.5
65	61.5
81	40.2
112	21.5
187	13.5

[a] Average of four values of specific activity

(5, 24, 38, 50 mCi/mg))

This means value has been assumed as 100 % value.

as reported by many other authors for other monoclonal antibodies. The availability of a high specific activity and stable material, labelled with either ^{131}I or ^{123}I, allowed its easy conversion to a sterile, pyrogenfree material, to be safely administered to patients, according to a well defined protocol (21) (23) (26).

The main problem of the F(ab')$_2$ labelling with ^{111}In, following the well known method of Hnatowich (20), was associated with the safe introduction of a chelating agent in the protein chain, achieving in the same time a maximum yield, an acceptable impairment of immunoreactivity and a minimum formation of aggregates.

After the conjugation of F(ab')$_2$ with DTPA, the molecular weight of the fragment and the presence of the aggregate form was checked by gel filtration on HPLC. As it is illustrated in Fig. 2 and confirmed by the data reported in Fig. 3, the peak of $F(ab')_2$-DTPA was eluted after intact IgB.

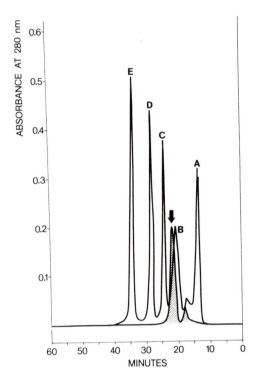

Figure 2.

Elution profile of a mixture of different proteins by gel filtration on HPLC. The column TSK G3000 was equilibrated with 0.05 M, pH 7.0 phosphate buffer, containing 0.3 M NACl and 0.05% sodium azide. The flow rate was 0.8 ml/min. The eluted peaks were : A. Human thyrolgobulin (hTG), B. Human immunoglobulin

(IgG), C. Ovoalbumin, D. Myoglobin, E. Vitamin B12.

The arrow shows the peak of F(ab')$_2$-DTPA.

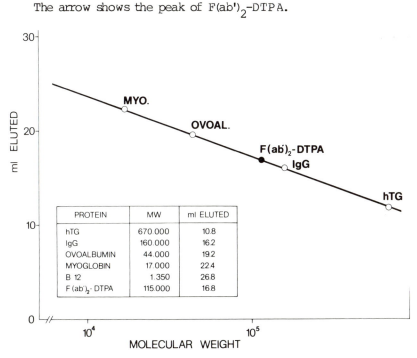

Figure 3.

Evaluation of the molecular weight of F(ab')$_2$-DTPA. In the table the molecular weights (MW) of the proteins used as a standard and the elution volume for each protein are reported.

The amount of aggregated F(ab')$_2$ was around 10%. The molecular weight of F(ab')$_2$-DTPA conjugate was found to be 115.000 daltons, as evaluated by performing HPLC analysis of a standard mixture of purified proteins at known molecular weight (human Thyroglobulin, human IgG, Ovoalbumin, Myoglobin and Vitamin B12), to which F(ab')$_2$-DTPA conjugate was added (Fig.3).

111

E

The availability of a stable conjugate, which can be stored at $-20^\circ C$ for several months, allows the ^{111}In-labelling step to be performed easily in a separate run, to be repeated at definite intervals according to the need. The yield of this second step of the process is very high, thus simplifying the purification problems and the quality control of the final labelled reagent.

All the radiotracer preparations were also evaluated by HPLC in order to check the reproducibility of the different ^{111}In tracer lots used for the clinical studies (26) (27) (28).

The preliminary results obtained in-vivo with ^{131}I and confirmed later with other radioisotopes have clearly shown a very early uptake of the radiolabelled $F(ab')_2$ by the tumour tissues. This finding, probably peculiar to the monoclonal antibody 225.28S, prompted us to study the possibility of ^{99m}Tc-labelling in order to develop an instant labelling procedure, as achieved for most of the Tc-labelled scintigraphic agents.

The direct Tc-labelling of $F(ab')_2$ by the pretinning procedure, already adopted by us in the past for other Tc-labelled proteins developed in our laboratories, was chosen also in this case, obtaining both an high labelling yield and a satisfactory in-vitro binding to target cells Colo 38, even after lyophlization of the reagents.

Having assessed the possibility of preparing an instant kit, most of our studies have concerned the development of safe quality control procedures, capable to check the purity of the final product and the reproducibility of different labelling runs.

The stability of the lyophilized $F(ab')_2$ prior to labelling has been investigated first. Data accumulated on a consistent number of lots have demonstrated that, when stored at $4^\circ C$, freeze-dried $F(ab')_2$, suitably conditioned in sterile penicillin bottles, can be safely labelled with ^{99m}Tc for at least 3-4 months without any significant loss of immunoreactivity in the tagged material.

The radiochemical purity test carried out by cellulose acetate electrophoresis, 5 hours after the labelling run, showed no relevant peak of ^{99m}Tc-labelled HSA in the final product (Fig. 4).

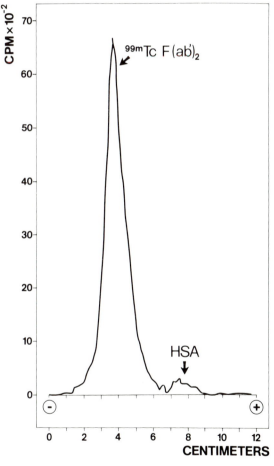

Figure 4.
Evaluation of radiochemical purity of ^{99m}Tc F(ab')₂ by

cellulose acetate electrophoresis, 5 hours after the labelling run. No significant radioactivity is associated with to HSA.

This demonstrated that the HSA used a proteic carrier in the lyophilization process was not Tc-labelled during the reaction with ^{99m}Tc-pertechnetate nor any significant exchange of Technetium occurred later between F(ab')$_2$ and HSA.

The purity of ^{99m}Tc-labelled F(ab')$_2$ from free ^{99m}Tc, was evaluated by gel chromatography on Biogel P6, at different times after labelling (Fig. 5).

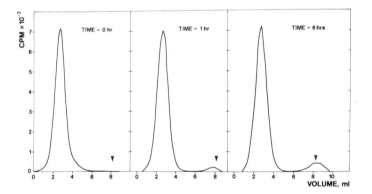

Figure 5.

Evaluation of radiochemical purity of ^{99m}Tc F(ab')$_2$ by Biogel

P6 gel chromatography.

Free Tc is evaluated at t = 0, 1 hr, 6 hrs after labelling and purification process.

Unbound Technetium, undetectable after purification of labelled material, increased to non relevant amounts after 1 hour (time suggested for the in-vivo administration of the radiotracer) and reached 5-8% after 6 hours.

The amount of Technetium released from the final product could not be significantly correlated with the kind of anionic resin column used for the separation of unbound from protein-bound Tc after the labelling process; however, a weaker anionic resin like DEAE Sephadex A-25 seemed to be slightly more effective. The choice of the resin was also strongly affected by its possibility to be properly conditioned and stored as sterile and pyrogen-free material. As a matter of fact, the availability of ready-to-use reagents largely simplifies the quality control, the shipment and the final handling of the material, provided that suitable care has been taken in the preparation of the reagents.

CONCLUSIONS

As the main objective of our work was the preparation of radiopharmaceutical grade reagents (both IgG and F(ab')₂ fragments) for in-vivo immunodetection of tumours, it may be considered substantially reached. Four different radionuclides, with different physical characteristics in terms of half life and radiation energy, have been safely employed, still keeping the immunoreactivity of the radiotracers at a substantially high level.

The particular feature of the anti-melanoma MoAb 225.28S 8i.e. early uptake by the tumour tissues) have rendered possible and feasible labelling with an ideal nuclide such as ^{99m}Tc.

In any case, the model of "experimental protocol" we have followed with substantially good results will constitute the basis for future studies to be carried out with other monoclonal antibodies and/or their $F(ab')_2$ and Fab fragments.

REFERENCES

1. Goldenberg D.M. Immunodiagnosis and immunodetection of colorectal cancer.

Cancer Bull. 30, 213-218, 1978.

2. Mach J.P., Carrel S., Forni M., Ritschard J., Donath A. and Alberto P. Tumour localization of radiolabelled antibodies against carcinoembryonic antigen in patients with carcinoma.

N. Eng. J. Med. 303, 5-10, 1980.

3. Deland F.H., Kim E.E., Simmions G. and Goldenberg D.M. Imaging approach in radioimmunodetection.

Cancer Res. 40, 3046-3049, 1980.

4. Primus F.J., MacDonald R., Goldenberg D.M. and Hansen H.J. Localization of GW-39 human tumours in hamsters by affinity-purified antibody to carcinoembryonic antigen.

Canc. Res. 37, 1544-1547, 1977.

5. Mach J.P., Buchegger F., Forni M., Ritschard J., Berche C., Lumbroso J.D., Schreyer M., Girardet C., Accolla L.S. and Carrel S. Use of radiolabelled monoclonal anti CEA antibodies for the detection of human carcinoma by external photoscanning and tomoscintigraphy.

Immunol. Today 2, 239-269, 1981.

6. Epenetos A.A., Britton K.E., Mather S., Shepherd J., Granowska M., Taylor-Papadimitriou J., Nic C.A., Durbin H., Hawkins L.R., Malpes J.S. and Bodmer W.F. Targeting of Iodine-123-labelled associated monoclonal antibodies to ovarian,

breast and gastro-intestinal tumours.

Lancet, ii, 999-1004, 1982.

7. Larson S.M., Brown J.P., Wright P.W., Carrasquillo J.A., Hellstrom I. and Hellstrom K.F. Imaging of melanoma with ^{131}I labelled monoclonal antibodies.

J. Nucl. Med. 24, 123-129, 1982.

8. Wilson B.S., Imai K., Natali P.G. and Ferrone S. Distribution and molecular characterization of a cell-surface and cytoplasmic antigen detectable in human melanoma cells with monoclonal antibodies.

Int. J. Cancer 28, 293-300, 1981.

9. Wilson B.S., Giacvomini P., Imai K., Natali P.G., Nakanishi T., Ruberto G. and Ferrone S. Human melanoma-associated antigens identified with monoclonal antibodies.

La Ricerca in Clinica e Laboratorio: XII (4), 517-538, 1984.

10. Natali P.G., Cavaliere R., Matsui M., Buraggi G., Callegaro L. and Ferrone S. Human melanoma associated antigen identified with monoclonal antibodies: characterization and potential clinical application. In "Cutaneous melanoma and procursor lesions" Ruiter D.J. Welvaart K. and Ferrone S. Eds. Martinus Nijhoff publishers 19-37, 1984.

11. Mariani G., Callegaro L., Mazzucca N., Cecconato E., Molea N., Dovis M., Fusani L., Deleide G., Buraggi G.L. and Bianchi R.

Tissue distribution of radiolabelled anti-CEA monoclonal antibodies in man. In "Protides in biological fluids" H. Peters Ed., Pergamon Press Vol. 32 (in press).

12. Buraggi G.L., Callegaro L., Turrin A., Gennari L., Bombardieri E., Gasparini M., Mariani G., Doci R., Regalia E. and Seregni E. Immunoscintigraphy of colorectal carcinoma: remarks

about an ongoing clinical trial.

Eur. J. Nucl., 1984 (In press).

13. Mazauric T., Mitchell K.F., Letchworth J.G., Koprowski H. and Steplewski Z. Monoclonal antibody-defined human lung cell surface protein antigens.

Cancer Res. 42, 150,154, 1982.

14. Boniolo A., Dovis M. and Matteja R. Use of an enzyme-linked immunosorbent assay for screening hybridoma antibodies against hepatitis B surface antigen.

J. Immunol. Meth. 49, 1-15, 1982.

15. Russo C., Callegaro L., Lanza E. and Ferrone S. Purification of IgG monoclonal antibody by caprylic acid precipitation.

J. Immunol. Meth. 65, 269-271, 1983.

16. Nisonoff A., Wissler F.C. and Woernley D.L. Properties of univalent fragments of rabbit antibody isolated by specific absorption.

Arch. Biochem. 88, 241-255, 1960.

17. Callegaro L., Ferrone S., Plassio G., Dovis M., Mariani G., Buraggi G.L., Boniolo A. and Rosa U. Biochemical characterization of monoclonal antibodies and F(ab')$_2$ fragment against human melanoma associated antigen labelled with different radioactive isotopes.

J. Nucl. Med. All. Sci. 27, 82-85, 1983.

18. Weber K. and Osborn M. The reliability of molecular weight determination by dodecyl sulphate-polyacrylamide gel electrophoresis.

J. Biol. Chem. 244, 4406-4412, 1969.

19 Salacinski P., Hope J., and McLean C. Iodination of proteins, glycoproteins and peptides using a solid phase oxidizing

agent (Iodo-Gen).

Anal. Biochem. 117, 136–146, 1981.

20. Knatowich D.J., Layne W.W. and Childs R.C. The preparation and labelling of DTPA–coupled albumin.

Int. J. Appl. radiat. Isot. 33, 327–332, 1982.

21. Buraggi G.L., Callegaro L., Mariani G., Turrin A., Cascinelli N., Attili A., Bombardieri E., Terno G., Plassio G., Dovis M., Mazzucca N., Natali P.G., Scassellati G.A., Rosa U. and Ferrone S.

Imaging with ^{131}I-labelled monoclonal antibodies to a high molecular weight-melanoma associated antigen in patients with melanoma: efficancy of whole Ig and its F(ab')$_2$ fragments.

Submitted for publication 1984.

22. Burchiel S.W., Khraw B.A., Rhodes B.A., Smith T.W. and Haber E. Immunopharmacokinetics of radiolabelled antibodies and their fragments in tumour imaging. The radiochemical detection of Cancer.

Burchiel S.W. and Rhodes B.A. Eds.

Masson Publishing U.S.A. Inc. 13, 125–139, 1982.

23. Mariani G., Callegaro L., Mazzucca N., Mencacci S., Ferrone S., Rosa U. and Bianchi R. In vivo distribution of antimelanoma monoclonal antibodies.

In "Protides in biological fluids" H. Peters Ed., Pergamon Press, Vol. 31, 971–976 (1984).

24. Gose T., Ferrone S., Imal K., Norwell S.T., Luner S.J., Marin R.H. and Blair A.H. Imaging of human melanoma xenografts in nude mice with a radiolabelled monoclonal antibody.

J. Natl. Cancer Inst. 69, 823–826, 1982.

25. Natali P.G., Giacomini P., Buraggi G.L., Cavaliere R., Bigotti A., Callegaro L. and Ferrone S.

Serological and binding characteristics of a monoclonal antibody (MoAb) to a human high molecular weight-melanoma associated antigen (HMW-MAA) for tumour imaging. In 6th International Symposium on Research in Tumour Immunology. Anacapri May 4-5, 1984.

26. Ferrone S., Giacomini P., Natali P.G., Ruiter D., Buraggi G.L. Callegaro L. and Rosa U. A human high molecular weight-melanoma associated antigen (HMW-MAA) defined by monoclonal antibodies: a useful marker to radioimage tumour lesions in patients with melanoma. In Proceedings of First International Meeting on Boron Neutron Capture M.I.T. Boston, October 12-14, 1983.

27. Buraggi G.L., Callegaro L., Turrin A., Cascinelli N., Attili A., Emanuelli H., Gasparini M., Deleide G., Plassio G., Dovis M., Mariani G., Natali P.G., Scassellati G.A., Rosa U. and Ferrone S. Immunoscintigraphy with ^{123}I, ^{99m}Tc and ^{111}In-labelled F'(ab')$_2$ fragments of monoclonal antibodies to a human high molecular weight-melanoma associated antigen (HMW-MAA). J. Nucl. Med. All. Sci. (in press).

28. Buraggi G.L., Callegaro L., Ferrone S., Turrin A., Cascinelli A., Attili A., Bombardieri E., Mariani G. and Deleide G. In Vivo immunodiagnosis with radiolabelled antimelanoma antibodies and F(ab')$_2$ fragments. Nuklear Medizin : Proceedings of the 21th Int. Ann. Meet. SNME Ulm 13-16 Sept. 1983. Ed. Schattauer Verlag Stuttgart, N.Y., 713-716, 1984.

Nuclear and other intracellular Organelles for Radionuclidic Tumour targeting: New Perspectives.

Hazra D.K. and Shabd Saran.

Nuclear Medicine and RIA Unit, Postgraduate Dept of Medicine. S.N. Medical College. Agra-282005 India.

SUMMARY

The use of intracellular targets for radionuclidic labelled antibody or other probes is analysed in relation to the limitations of cell surface targeting, the choice of intracellular target (Oncogene, Z-DNA, mitochondria, plasmids etc.) or related growth factors or growth factor receptors and methods of effecting intracellular entry particularly the possible use of Fc receptors, liposomes, hybrid immunoglobulins and hemi-immunoglobulins.

INTRODUCTION

The contemporary explosion of interest in monoclonal antibodies has led to their use being explored in various fields. We have reviewed elsewhere (1 and 2), the scope of monoclonal antibodies in oncology and in particular the use of radionuclidic labelled antibodies in tumour targeting both for radioimmuno-imaging as well as for radioimmunotherapy. We had suggested the possible use of intracellular targets for these labelled antibodies, in particular, nuclear and mitochondrial targets (1,3). Recent methodological advances and clearer understanding of the intracellular changes in cancer allow one to postulate the problems and potential of this approach in greater detail and this is the subject of the present communication.

LIMITATIONS OF SHED ANTIGENS AND CELL SURFACE ANTIGENS AS TARGETS

The early work on cancer detection by in vitro assay of tumours associated products in the blood or other body fluids of cancer patients led to the emphasis on circulating shed antigens such as carcinoembryonic antigen (CEA), Alfafeto-protein (AFP) and human chorionic gonadotropin (HCG). It was perhaps natural and inevitable that the availability of antisera for in vitro measurement of tumour marker antigens led to their being used for in vivo tumour targeting.

This approach was intrinsically limited by the fact that the circulating shed antigen would compete with the same antigen located in the tumour for an administered antibody. However, Rhodes et al. (4) who developed an animal model with hCG immobilized on sepherose beads, found that using Tc^{99m} labelled Fab_2 fragments, the uptake of the antibody to the solid phase hCG sepharose implant was not affected by circulating hCG. This experiment suggests that at least in this model antibody fragment localization at sites of immobile antigen is not inhibited by circulating antigens.

It was also apparent from in vitro diagnostic studies that the common shed antigens were not even tumour specific. For example serum CEA levels are raised in many non-malignant colonic lesions. Mach observed that using radio-labelled antibodies against CEA whether polyclonal or monoclonal, only 0.1% of the administered antibody localized in the tumour (5). This was a serious limitation for therapy and even for imaging because of the high blood background. Several dual scanning techniques were, therefore, adopted to permit subtraction of the blood background. Temporal subtraction (6) of early from late images or of one isotope imaging the blood background from another isotope following the antibody distribution (7) would salvage radioimmuno-detection (although here too there were technical problems (8)), but this subtraction would obviously not be of help in achieving specific radioimmunotherapy.

The next step forward was the use of cell surface fixed antigens such as $HFMG_2$ receptor. This greatly increased the fraction of radioactivity localizing in the tumour (9). However, the general problems of targeting surface antigens remain formidable.

The phenomenon of antigenic modulation is well recognized (10). Tumour cells exhibiting a surface antigen tend to alter this expression when exposed to antibody, thus rendering the latter ineffective. Even without the presence of antibodies tumour cells show variation in surface antigens from time to time. Also a tumour may contain two or more populations of cells each of which has a different surface antigens (11). Surface antigens may also differ between the parent tumour and its metastases (12). Using monoclonal antibody immunohistochemical techniques Fabr and Daar (1984) have demonstrated that tumours are very hetrogenous with respect to cell surface markers and that this may be related to biological behaviour of the tumour (13). Further, the surface properties of tumour arising from the same tissue can vary widely for example the slow and rapid growing varieties of the Morris heptomas (12).

The cell surface antigens of tumour cell lines in vitro can also depart considerably from those of the parent tumour (14). It is known that chemically induced tumours have antigens related primarily to the carcinogens and quite different from those of spontaneous tumours. This considerably limits the use of such cell lines or experimental tumours for raising or testing presumptive anti-tumour antibodies.

One approach to the multiplicity of the surface antigens is to use an 'engineered cocktail' of monoclonal antibodies directed against such antigens, but one can not be certain of targeting all the surface antigens. Cell surface changes are secondary to the basic malignant change in the nucleus. Similarly metabolic changes can also be related to the changes in the genes (15). Targeting the malignant nuclei is similar to modern warfare techniques where enemy capitals are destroyed by guided missiles rather than skirmishes at frontiers! These considerations suggest that our hypothesis of using intracellular targets for antibody mediated attack is increasingly relevant.

CHOICE OF INTRACELLULAR TARGETS

1. About a decade ago our knowledge of the nuclear changes in cancer cells was very limited. Large number of mitotic figure in tumour tissues as well as occurrence of chromosomal deletions, translocations and aneuploidy were known but even the most recognized nuclear change i.e. the presence of Philadelphia chromosome in Chronic Granulocytic Leukaemia (CGL) was not observed in all cases.

We have come a long way since than. Recently it has been reported by Sincock that it is possible to recognise not only malignant cells but also premalignant cells by virtue of their greater quantities of new DNA by Feulgen staining (16). However, this approach would fail if one also considers rapidly growing normal tissues of intestinal epithelia.

2. The study of tumour viruses led to the recognitition of small number of viral nucleotides fragments in cancer cells and these viral sequences were labelled as viral oncogenes. Gene

isolation techniques from human cancers and from human non-cancerous cells based on their ability to transform NIH - 3T3 cells in vitro by transfection led to the identification of a number of nucleotide sequences homologous to the viral oncogenes and these were termed proto-oncogenes (17-19). It was later observed that these cellular proto-oncogenes can also be oncogenic.

The mechanism by which retro-virus oncogenes which are merely copies of normally existing cellular oncogenes as described above become carcinogenic has been studied. According to the dosage hypothesis the reason is merely the large quantity of a normally occurring cell protein under the stimulation by viral regulatory transcriptional sequences (17). Secondly the cellular oncogenes contain separate domains called exons with intervening regions known as introns. The cellular genes mos and ras lack transformation actitivy when associated with their normal cellular flanking sequences, but when translocated to new sites they become carcinogenic (20).

Another method by which the proto-oncogene becomes oncogenic has been discovered by Tabin (21) and Reddy (22). A point mutation occurs in the oncogene causing GC to TA transversion i.e. Guanine Cytosine is replaced by Thymidine Adenosine. This results in glycine being replaced by valine at the 12th position of the T_{24} oncogene encoded p^{21} protein. Valine has a bulky side chain unlike glycine which affects its interaction with cellular targets.

A fourth mechanism has also being identified. The erb-B gene creates an Epidermal growth Factor (EGF) receptor which is incomplete and lacks the control region that enables cellular replication to be shut off (23). It is noteworthy that certain brain tumours contain high concentrations of EGF receptor and it has also been reported that the EGF receptor is associated with an endonuclease which acts directly on DNA. Like DNA topo-isomerase II, this EGF receptor can nick double stranded circular DNA in the presence of ATP (24). Such mechanisms may result in abnormal stimulation of the DNA and cell division.

Abnormal cellular multiplication due to enhanced production of a protein coded by the sis oncogen similar to normal platelet derived growth factor (PDGF) has been hypothesized (25,26).

3. Thus oncogenes, associated growth factors and growth factor receptors appear logical targets for designing immunological warheads. If the dosage hypothesis is accepted the malignant cells will have a greater quantity of these epitopes, as compared to normal cells. If in addition, there are alterations in structure (e.g. proto-oncogene to oncogene, normal cell protein to abnormal cell protein, normal receptor to abnormal receptor), it may be possible to design antisera that specifically recognise these alteration.

4. There have been several reports on the occurrence of left handed Z-DNA instead of the normal double helix in malignant cells. It is also possible to raise antisera which recognise abnormal Z-DNA (27). Whether these can be applied to intracellulr targeting merits exploration.

5. As contrasted to the bewildering surfeit of surface antigens in cancer cells, it is heartening to note that 'fewer and fewer' oncogenes - about a score are now believed to be of significance (18). Thus they constitute a limited number of targets as compared to the numerous surface antigens which will be logistically convenient for immunotherapy.

6. Apart from oncogenes, growth factors and Z-DNA the growth factor receptor targeting is specially attractive. The antibody will (a) interfere with response to growth factor and (b)

126

if armed with a radioactive warhead, it may destroy the tumour cell bearing this receptor. Mroczkowski et al. have reported high levels of this receptor in cancer cells under the control of oncogene erb-B (24). Growth factor receptor are located at least partially at the cell surface conveniently exposed to antibody attack. They may also offer a mechanism for the internalization of the receptor-linked antibody.

7. We have also conceived of mitochondria of cancer cells as targets (1,3). The mitochondria are the major seats of energy transformation in the cell. The known metabolic differences between normal and malignant cells for exaple the preferential anaerobic metabolism and critical dependence on glucose suggests that there may be structural antigenic differences in the mitochondria present in cancer cells vis a vis normal cells.

Mitochondria have been regarded as renants of once independent organisms which parasitized in the cells. It has been hypothesized that in tumours owing to mutation the mitochondrion loses its symbiotic relationship with the nuceus and starts replicating at the expense of the cell. Hartung from New York has suggested that mitochondrial DNA is more liable to mutation and less capable of repair as compared to nuclear DNA because it is not bound to protective proteins and he has suggested that the continuous mitoses of the cancer cells are unsuccessful attempts to get rid of the mutant mitochondria (28).

The possibility of mitochondrial mutation as well as the recognition of altered metabolism in cancer cells both suggest the existance of distinctive mitochondrial epitopes in malignant cells as compared to normal cells.

8. Human plasmids have been recently discovered by Clabrettea et al. (29). These are small loops of DNA outside the

nucleus. They may represent retro-viruses. Flavell et al. working on the fruitfly, Drosophila found that plasmids are derived from the mobile genetic element copia and also resembles an avian Retro-vituses (3 @). If abnormal human plasmids are found to be widely distributed in human cancer cells, they also may be targeted. Antibodies directed against such extra-nuclear DNA need not cross the second barrier of the nuclear membrane thus further simplifying targeting.

THE PROBLEM OF INTRACELLULAR ENTRY

No attempts appear to have been made to target intra-cellular antigens because it was thought that antibodies can not cross the cell membrane. Several consideration, however, lead us to believe that intracellular targeting is possible.

1. The occurrence of antinuclear antibodies in systemic lupus erythematosus (SLE) has long been documented, but it was not certain as to whether these are pathogenic entering living cells or whether they merely represent post hoc phenomenon in response to liberated nuclear protein.

However, Segovia et al. have shown that antinuclear ribonuclear protein can penetrate life T suppressor cells via the Fc receptor and destroy their suppressor function suggesting that his antibody activity is not a laboratory artifact (31).

2. The transcellular transport of immunoglobulins across lining epithelia and heptocytes involves receptor mediated uptake with subsequent reappearance and release of ligand at the cell surface (32,33). This is again an example of the entry of immunoglobulins into living cells. Certain proteins remain attached to the limiting membrane of the endosome and are routed out of the cell surface-lysosome pathway (34). Antibody mediated surface receptor

aggregation appears to be a very important phenomenon (35).

Fc receptor mediated intracellular transport would not apply, however, to labelled Fab and Fab_2 fragments which are being currently evaluated because of their smaller non-specific uptake by the reticulo-endothelial system (RES).

3. Secondly we suggest that the cellular entry may be facilitated in tumour cells as compared to normal cells and especially so during cell division when the cell membrane is stretched and thinned out. Teleradiotherapy may be used to further enhance the cellular permeability. For superficial lesions the effect of laser or ultrasound on cellular permeability needs exploration.

4. Using antibodies directed against intracellular tissue polypeptide antigens associated with keratin, there have been reports of successful imaging in animal models (36). If these reports are confirmed, the possibility of targeting other intracellular and mitochondrial antigens is strengthened.

5. It has recently become possible to synthesize hybrid monoclonal immunoglobulins in which the two halves of the immunoglobulin molecule recognize different antigenic sites (37). The possibility, therefore, arises of devising hybrid immuno-globulins one arm of which is directed against a surface antigen while the other looks at an intracellular nuclear or mitochondrial antigen (38).

6. Spontaneously occurring hybridoma mutants sometimes gnerate hemi-immunoglobulin molecules whose properties are of great interest (39). These do not bond to Fc receptors and also do not aggregate or modulate tumour antigens. Whether these can penetrate living cells using modes other than Fc receptors, needs to be determined.

The surface antigen which mediates internalization of the antibody need not be 100% tumour specific. It may even be shared by normal and malignant cells of a particular tissue but the intracellular antigen must be one that is distinctive for tumour cells.

7. It is also possible to enter intact cells through a Trojan horse approach – the antibody may be encapsulated in a liposome. Anti-RNA has been introduced using liposomes into adenovirus type II infected Hela cells and this successfully altered the expression of the adeno-virus genes, inhibiting the editing out of the introns (40).

8. Other approaches to intracellular entry may also be discussed here. Lections have been used as cell surface probes and have been labelled with Fluorochromes, Ferritin or radio-ligands. Many lectins are mitogenic, in addition animal lectins have been postulated to have intracellular functions apart from their surface functions and therefore, must need enter living cells (41,42). Since lectins can recognize carbohydrate antigens like antibodies, they can also conceivably be used to target intracellular structures.

9. Hormones such as corticosteroids or radiolabelled nucleotides such as I^{125} – IUDR(43) have been studied as possible intra-cellular probes. DNA hybrid probes have been used for in vitro identification of DNA sequences but this approach has been applied to digested cellular material and not to intact living cells. Extreme caution may be required before DNA fragments are introduced in vivo in human subjects.

CONCLUSIONS

It appears increasingly likely that intracellular nuclei, mitochondria or other intracellular organelles will be exploited as targets for immunlogical probes in vivo. Although scepticism has been expressed regarding the recognition by the immune response of oncogenes (44), these oncogenes, associated growth factors and growth factor receptors will obviously be evaluated in detail. The problem of interiorization on intact antibodies into living cells for immunotherapy using radionuclidic or other warheads may not be insoluble and some approaches have been suggested for evaluation.

ACKNOWLEDGEMENT

We are thankful to Dr. John Roder of Queen's University, Canada regarding Hybrid immunoglobulins discussion.

REFERENCES

1. Hazra D.K. and Sharma R.C. Nuclear Medicine Communications 1982; 3:210.

2. Hazra D.K. and Dass S. Current Science 1984; 53:842.

3. Hazra D.K. Lahiri V., Saran S et al. International Symposium on Immunoscintigraphy. Ivalo (Saariselka), Lapland, August 1984.

4. Rhodes B.A., Burke D.J. Breslow K. et al. Effect of circulating antigen on antibody localization in vivo : Radio-immunoimaging and Radioimmunotherapy 1983 ed. Ed. Burchiel S.W. and Rhodes B.A. Elsevier, New York, pp25.

5. Mach J.P. Forni M., Ritschard J. et al. Oncodevelop. Biol. Med. 1980, 1:49.

6. Granowska M., Britton K.E. and Shepherd J., Radiobiol. Radiother. 1984, 25:153.

7. Goldenberg D.M. Deland F., Kim E. et al New eng. J. Med., 1978, 298:1385.

8. Begent R.M.J., Stanway G., Jones B.E. et al. J. Royal Soc. Med. 1980, 73:624.

9. Epenetos A.A., Britton K.E. Mather S. et al. Lancet 1982,II:999.

10. Ritz J., Schlossman S.F. Utilization of monoclonal antibodies in the treatment of Leukemia and lymphoma. Review Blood 1982; 59:1.

11. Epenetos, A.A., Personal communication, 1984.

12. Sherbet G.V. The biology of Tumour Malignancy. Academic Press, London, New York, 1982, pp66.

13. Fabr. J.W. and Daar A.S. Expression of normal epithelial membrane antigens on human colorectal and breast carcinomas ; Radioimmunoimaging and Radioimmunotherapy. Ed. Burchiel S.W. and Rhodes B.A., Elsevier New York, ed. 1982, pp. 143.

14. Bale W.F. Contreras M.A. and Grady E.D. Cancer Res. 1980, 40:2965.

15. Weber G. Cancer Res. 1982, 43:3466.

16. Sincock A. Precancerous cells object of study. Quoted by Wright P. in the Statesman, New Delhi, Sept. 5, 1984, pp.9.

17. Cooper G.M. Science 1982, 217:801.

18. Weinburg R.A. Cell 1982, 30:3.

19. Hamlyn P. and Sikora K. Lancet 1983, II:326.

20. Rechavi G., Givol D. and Cannani E. Nature (London) 1982, 300:607.

21. Tabin D.J., Bradley S.M. Bargmann C.I. and Weinberg R.A. Nature (London) 1982, 300:143.

22. Reddy E.P. et al. Nature (London) 1982, 300:149.

23. Hayman M.J. and Beng H. Nature (London) 1984, 309:460.

24. Mroczkowki B., Mosig G. and Cohen S. Nature (London) 1984, 309:270.

25. Doolittle, R.F., Hunkapiller M.W. Devare S.G. et al. Science 1984, 221:275.

26. Waterfield M.D., Scrace G.T., Whittle N. et al. Nature (London) 1983, 304:35.

27. Lafer E.M., Möller A., Nordheim A et al. Proc. Natl. Acad. Sci. U.S.A. 1981, 781:3546.

28. Hartung J. Jr. Theor. Biol. 1982, 94:173.

29. Calabretta B., Robberson D.L. Barrera-Saldana H.A. et al. Nature (London) 1982, 296:219.

30. Flavell A.J. and Ish-Horowiez D. Nature (London) 1981, 292:591.

31. Alarcon-Segovia D., Ruiz-Arguelles A. and Llorent L. J. Immunol. 1979, 122:1855.

32. Renston R.H. et al, Science 1980, 208:1276.

33. Rodewald R.J. Cell Biol. 1980, 85:18.

34. Hopkins C.R. Nature 1983, 304:634.

35. King A.C. and Cuatrecasas P. The New Eng. J. Med. 1981, 305:77.

36. Winkler C., Oehr P. Roent trends in Radioimmunodetection of tumour. Presented at 2nd International Symposium on Human Tumour Markers, Vienna, 1984. Personal communication from Burchella J. and Lane E.B.

37. Milstein C. and Cuello A.C. Nature (London) 1983, 305:537.

38. Hazra D.K. and Saran Shabd. Current Science 1984 (In press).

39. Pollock R.R. Metlay J., Thammana P. et al. Generation of mutant Monoclonal Antibodies with changes in Biologic Function : Radioimmunoimaging and Radioimmunotherapy. Ed Burchiel S.W. and Rhodes B.A., Elsevier, New York, 1983, pp. 93.

40. Yang V.W., Lerner M.R., Steitz J.A., et al. Proc. Natl. Acad. Sci. 1981, 78:1371.

41. Barondes S.H. Ann. Rev. Biochem. 1981, 50:207.

42. Noujaim A.A., Shysh A., Bray Z.J. et al. Thomsen-Friendenreich Antigen : Radioimmunoimaging and Radioimmunotherapy. Ed. Burchiel S.W. and Rhodes B.A., Elsevier, New York, 1983, pp. 277.

43. Adelstein S.J., Feindegen L.E. Fowler J.F., Jentzsch K. and Kaercher K. Radiotion Biology of Auger Emitters and their therapeutic application. IAEA Consultant Report 1976.

44. Klein E. Biological Basis of Tumour Markers : Impact of the recent developments in the oncogene field on tumour immunology. 2nd International Conference on Tumour Markers, Vienna, Abstract 001, 1984.

Radioimmunodetection of Human Tumour Xenografts by Monoclonal Antibodies Correlates with antibody Density and Affinity[1]

Powe J.[2], Herlyn D.[3], Alavi A.[4], Munz D.[3],
Steplewski Z.[3] and Koprowski H.[3]

[1]This work was supported in part by grants CA-25874, CA-21124, and CA-10815, from the National Cancer Institute and the National Institutes of Health.

[2] Dr. J. Powe, Department of Nuclear Medicine, Victoria Hospital, London, Ontario, Canada N6A 4G5.

Work performed while a Fellow of the Medical Research Council of Canada at The Wistar Institute, Philadelphia, PA.

[3]The Wistar Institute of Anatomy and Biology, Philadelphia, PA 19104.

[4]Division of Nuclear Medicine, Hospital of the University of Pennsylvania, Philadelphia, PA 19104.

INTRODUCTION

The localization of human tumour exnografts in mice by radiolabelled monoclonal antibodies (MAbs) has met, in general, with success (1-10). However, poor tumour localization of some of the labelled antibody preparations is also observed (11,12), and the presence of circulating tumour antigens with the formation of immune complexes (11,13), and rapid degradation of antibody molecules by the tumour cells (12) have been examined as possible explanation for this failure. We have previously reported the successful imaging of human colorectal carcinoma (CRC) xenografts in immunosuppressed mice by two anti-CRC MAbs and have demonstrated that localization was enhanced when $F(ab')_2$ fragments were used instead of intact immunoglobulin (9). In the present study, we selected several anti-melanoma MAbs from a large panel available (14-19), and examined the ability of their ^{131}I-labelled $F(ab')_2$ fragments to radioimage human tumour xenografts in nude mice. Some of the MAbs successfully localized tumours, while others directed against the same tumour did not. The answer to the question of why some anti-tumour MAbs effectively locate tumours in vivo whereas others do not is of importance for the selection of MAbs which may be of use in radioimaging human tumours.

MATERIALS AND METHODS

Human Tumour Cell Lines

The melanoma cell line WM9 and the CRC cell lines SW948 and SW1222 have been described elsewhere (20, 21). These cell lines are maintained in culture in our laboratory.

Mice and Xenografts

Four to six week old nude mice (nu/nu BALB/c background) were injected subcutaneously with 1.5 x 10' human tumour cells either in the dorsal region or left flank. Beginning 48 hours before antibody administration, all mice were given 0.1% (W/V) KI in the drinking water to block thyroid uptake of free radioiodine. Some of the data obtained with anti-CRC MAbs CO 2032 and CO 17-1A were derived from xenografted immunosuppressed mice as previously described (9).

Murine MAbs

The eight anti-tumour MAbs (6 anti-melanoma and 2 anti-CRC) used in these experiments are described in Table 1. The anti-melanoma MAbs ME D63 and ME C44 bind to different determinants on the p97 antigen previously described by Woodbury et al. (23). Monoclonal anti-hepatitis virus antibody A5C3 (IgG2a) was used as a control antibody and was kindly supplied by Centocor, Malvern, PA.

Purification of MAbs and Production of F(ab')$_2$

MAbs were purified from ascitic fluid on Protein A-Sepharose columns as previously described (9). F(ab')$_2$ fragments were produced by pepsin digestion and purified using a Protein A-Sepharose column and chromatography on LKB Ultrogel AcA44 as described (9). All MAbs and F(ab')$_2$ preparations were checked for purity using sodium dodecyl sulfate-polyacrylamide gel electrophoresis.

137

TABLE 1

CHARACTERISTICS OF THE ANTI-TUMOUR MONOCLONAL ANTIBODIES EXAMINED

MAb Code	Isotype	Immunizing Tumor Type	Antigen Recognized (Molecular Weight)	Reference
ME 37-7	IgG2a	Melanoma	HLA-DR (38K, 31K, 28K)	16
ME 82-11	IgG1	Melanoma	NGF[a] receptor (75K)	14, 19
ME D63	IgG2a	Melanoma	Glycoprotein (97K)	17
ME 28-8	IgG2a	Melanoma	n.i.[b]	17
ME C44	IgG2a	Melanoma	Glycoprotein (97K)	17
ME 95-45	IgG1	Melanoma	Proteoglycan	14, 18
CO 17-1A	IgG2a	CRC	Protein, n.i.	21
CO 2032	IgG2a	CRC	Glycoprotein	22

[a] NGF = nerve growth factor

[b] n.i. = not identified

Radiolabelling of MAbs and F(ab')$_2$ Fragments

MAbs or their F(ab')$_2$ fragments were labelled with ^{125}I or ^{131}I using the Iodogen method as previously described (9). All in vitro assays were performed using ^{131}I or ^{125}I-labelled intact MAbs or F(ab')$_2$ fragments (specific activities 0.5 - 2.5 uCi/ug), whereas in vivo experiments were performed with ^{131}I or ^{125}I-labelled F(ab')$_2$ fragments only (2.0-5.0 uCi/ug).

In Vitro Antibody Binding Assays

Immunoreactivity and binding specificity of radiolabelled MAbs were determined in vitro prior to their use in tumour localization studies as described (9, 10, 24). Only preparations exhibiting > 70% immunoreactivity were used in the in vivo experiments. The maximal number of antibody binding sites per cell and the association constants (Ka) and MAb binding were determined by the methods of Scatchard (25) in binding assays described by us in detail elsewhere (17).

In Vivo Tissue Distribution of Radiolabelled MAbs and Radioimaging of Human Tumour Xenografts

^{131}I-labelled F(ab')$_2$ fragments were injected into mice bearing 7- to 10-day-old melanoma or CRC tumours weighing 70-150 mg. For tissue distribution studies, approximately 15 uCi of ^{131}I-labelled tumour-specific F(ab')$_2$ and 15 uCi of ^{125}O-labelled A5C3 control F(ab')$_2$ were simultaneously injected intraperitoneally. Two and four days later, the mice were sacrificed and the tumours and organs removed, blotted dry, weighed and assayed for radioactivity as previously described (9). Results are expressed as follows:

a) ratios of activity of specific $F(ab')_2$ in tumour tissue to that in normal mouse tissue <(cpm/mg tumour tissue)/(cpm/mg mouse tissue)>;

b) percentage of injected dose per gram of tissue, corrected for physical decay;

c) ratios of specific (^{131}I) to non-specific (^{125}I) activity in tumour divided by the same ratio in blood (4), i.e., the localization index.

For gamma-scintigraphy, mice bearing 7- to 9-day-old tumours received 100 uCi of ^{131}I labelled $F(ab')_2$ fragments, and images were obtained daily for up to 5 days as described previously (9). Images were visually graded using an arbitrary scale: (a) −, tumour not visualized; (b) +, tumour just discernable above background; (c) ++, clear but only fair visualization of tumour; and (d) +++, excellent tumour visualization.

Statistics

To determine whether in vitro binding correlated with in vivo tissue distribution of MAbs, the number of binding sites per cell and the association constant for each of the six anti-melanoma MAbs were expressed as natural logs (ln), summed and plotted against the ln of either % injected dose/g or the localiztion index, and the regression coefficient was calculated (26). WM9 was used as the target cell line. Significance of the correlation was analyzed by Student's t-test.

RESULTS

Radioimaging of Human Tumour Xenografts

Melanomas and CRC tumours could be clearly visualized by

gamma-scintigraphy in a large portion of xenotransplanted nude mice injected with ^{131}I-labelled F(ab')$_2$ fragments of either anti-melanoma MAb ME D63 or anti-CRC MAbs CO 17–1A and CO 2032, respectively (Table 2, Fig. 1), consistent with previously reported results (9, 10) on the basis of a much larger number of mice. Anti-melanoma MAbs ME 37–7 and ME 82–11, on the other hand, demonstrated poor tumour visualization in only 62% and 43% of the mice, respectively (Table 2, Fig 1). Three other anti-melanoma MAbs, ME 28–8, ME C44, and ME 94–45, did not visualize melanomas in any of the mice included for up to 5 days following the injection of the various MAbs (Table 2). Specificity of tumour localization by MAbs was confirmed by the absence of accumulation of ^{131}I-labelled control MAb to radioimage either melanoma or CRC xenografts in nude mice (not shown).

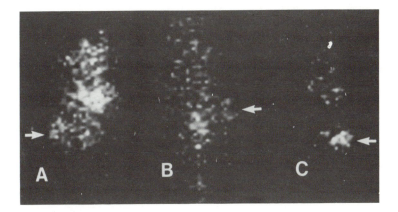

Figure 1

Gamma scintigraphy of human melanomas transplanted to nude mice 3–4 days after the injection of 100 uCi ^{131}I-labelled ME 37–7 F(ab')$_2$(A), ME 82–11 F(ab')$_2$(B), or ME D63 F(ab')$_2$(C). Seven to 10 days following MAb injection, the tumour xenotransplants were injected subcutaneously in the flank as indicated by arrows.

Table 2

RADIOIMAGING OF HUMAN TUMOUR XENOGRAFTS[a]

MAb	Target Cell Line	Fraction of Xenografts Visualized	Average Tumour Visualization Grade
ME 37-7	WM9	5/8	+
ME 82-11	WM9	5/16	+
ME D63	WM9	16/21	++
CO 17-1A	SW948	20/25	++
CO 2032	SW1222	4/4	+++
ME 28-8	WM9	0/5	−
ME C44	WM9	0/8	−
ME 95-45	WM9	0/5	−

[a] Four to 25 xenografted mice were imaged for 2–5 days after injection of 100 uCi ^{131}I-labelled F(ab')$_2$ (see Materials and Methods).

In Vivo Tissue Distribution of Radiolabelled MAb – F(ab')$_2$ Fragments

The specific activities of radiolabelled MAb F(ab')$_2$ fragments in tumour tissues xenografted onto mice were compared with the activities in normal mouse tissues. Tumour-to-tissue ratios of radioactivity were higher 4 days after the injection of ^{131}I-labelled F(ab')$_2$ than after 2 days (not shown). Tumour-to-tissue ratios for the radioimaging MAbs differed significantly ($p < 0.025$) from those of the control MAb for all tissues tested except for the tumour-to-kidney ratios obtained with

MAb 17-aA (Table 3).

TABLE 3

DISTRIBUTION OF RADIOLABELED MAb F(ab')₂ FRAGMENTS IN

HUMAN TUMOR GRAFTED NUDE MICE

Tumor Visualization by γ-Scintigraphy[a]	MAb	Tumor/Tissue Ratios of Radioactivity [(cpm/mg in tumor)/(cpm/mg in tissue)][b] TISSUE							Localization Index[b]
		Blood	Liver	Spleen	Kidney	Lung	Heart	Muscle	
POSITIVE	ME 37-7	10.9* ± 8.4	18.2* ± 6.0	35.5* ± 20.3	9.8* ± 4.1	8.4* ± 3.0	18.3 ± 9.1	62.2* ± 45.3	2.7* ± 1.0
	ME 82-11	17.7* ± 10.4	20.6 ±10.9	27.37*± 12.1	13.8* ± 6.4	13.2* ± 7.8	49.4* ± 34.6	101.3 ± 42.4	6.9* ± 3.8
	ME D63[c]	33.8* ± 8.7	84.2* ± 1.7	72.4* ± 26.8	46.5* ± 11.6	41.6* ± 10.6	119.6* ± 45.2	219.4* ± 97.8	15.9* ± 7.3
	CO 17-1A[c]	18.7* ± 6.8	6.7* ± 1.9	20.4* ± 9.5	3.6 ± 1.7	7.7* ± 4.3	26.0* ± 5.7	66.8* ± 26.7	7.6* ± 5.1
	CO 2032[c]	52.3* ± 15.4	57.8* ±11.3	87.3* ± 39.4	24.2* ± 6.1	30.4* ± 7.3	122.7* ± 53.2	215.4* ± 77.4	11.4* ± 5.3
NEGATIVE	ME 28-8	1.3 ± 0.3	2.6 ± 0.3	2.9 ± 0.5	0.7 ± 0.4	1.2 ± 0.3	3.9 ± 0.8	10.0 ± 2.1	0.9 ± 0.2
	ME C44	1.7 ± 0.4	6.0 ± 1.5	6.6 ± 1.7	2.7 ± 0.7	3.7 ± 0.9	8.5 ± 1.3	17.8 ± 3.3	0.9 ± 0.2
	ME 95-45	1.3 ± 0.7	9.3 ± 3.5	8.7 ± 3.8	4.2 ± 1.8	3.4 ± 1.0	6.9 ± 2.7	18.2 ± 6.4	0.7 ± 0.0/
	ASC3[d]	2.1 ± 1.1	2.8 ± 1.3	2.6 ± 1.8	1.4 ± 1.0	1.9 ± 1.0	8.9 ± 4.6	15.1 ± 10.0	n.d.

a Details are given in Table 2 and Fig. 1.

b Mean ± S.D. of 3-8 mice 4 days after the simultaneous injection of 15 Ci each of ¹³¹I-labeled specific F(ab')₂ and ¹²⁵I-labeled F(ab')₂ of control MAb ASC3.

c Results have been presented previously (9, 10).

d Values obtained with control MAb ASC3 did not differ for melanomas and CRC tumors and are therefore averaged for both tumor types.

* Values differ significantly (p < 0.05) from each of the values obtained with the non-radioimaging MAbs.

F

Furthermore, all but a few ratios obtained with each of the radioimaging MAbs were significantly (p < 0.05) higher than the ratios obtained with any of the non-radioimaging MAbs. Due to the high variability of the tumour-to-liver, tumour-to-heart and tumour-to-muscle ratios obtained in individual mice with the radioimaging MAbs 82-11 and 37-7, these ratios did not differ significantly (p > 0.05) from the corresponding ratios of some of the non-radioimaging MAbs (Table 3). Ratios for the radioimaging MAb ME D63 were significantly (p < 0.05) higher than those obtained with each of the other radioimaging anti-melanoma MAbs for all tissues examined and the values were on the order of magnitude previously reported for this MAb (10).

Finally, the tumour-to-tissue ratios obtained with $F(ab')_{2*}$ fragments of the non-radioimaging MAbs ME 28-8, ME C44 and ME 95-45 were not significantly (p > 0.05) different from those obtained with control A5C3 $F(ab')_2$, with the exception of the tumour-to-liver and tumour-to-spleen ratios obtained with MAbs ME C44 and ME 95-45 (Table 3).

Further evidence of specific localization of MAbs in tumour tissues was established by comparing the tumour and the blood distribution of ^{131}I-labelled specific MAb and ^{125}I-labelled control MAb injected simultaneously into tumour-bearing nude mice (Table 3). The localization indices derived from specific antibody-to-control antibody ratios in tumour tissue relative to blood were between 2.7 and 15.9 for the radioimaging MAbs, as compared with values of <1.0 for non-radioimaging MAbs. Accumulation of the radioimaging MAbs in tumour tissues relative to blood was significantly greater than that of control antibody and the localization indices were significantly higher (p <0.05)

144

than those of the non-radioimaging MAbs.

Since the ability of antibodies to localize tumours by external gamma-scintigraphy is dependent not only on the preferential binding of the antibodies to tumour tissues, but also on the specific activities of radioactivity accumulated in these tissues, the possibility was tested that radioimaging and non-radioimaging MAbs differ in their specific activities in tumour tissues. The percentage of antibody dose injected per g tumour tissue was significantly higher (p < 0.05) for each of the radioimaging MAbs as compared to any of the non-imaging MAbs (Table 4). Thus, radioimaging MAbs accumulated significantly higher amounts of radioactivity in the tumours than did the non-radioimaging MAbs.

Scatchard Analysis of In Vitro MAb Binding

To determine whether differences in binding reactivities to tumour cells account for the observation that radioimaging MAbs accumulate significantly higher amounts of radioactivity in tumour tissues as compared to non-radioimaging MAbs, the binding characteristics of MAbs to their specific target cells were analyzed in vitro by the method of Scatchard (25). Since iodination might conceivably affect the binding of MAbs to tumour cells, the results of both direct binding assays and inhibition assays were analyzed separately and compared as previously described (17). With both methods, nearly identical Ka values and maximum number of antibody molecules bound per cell were obtained for each of the eight MAbs included, suggesting that iodination did not significantly alter the binding of these MAbs. There was a wide range in Ka values ($0.1 - 83 \times 10^8$ M^{-1}) and in maximum number of molecules bound per cell ($0.07 - 5.4 \times 10^6$) (Table 4). No in vivo localization of radiolabelled anti-melanoma $F(ab')_2$

fragments was demonstrable for fewer than 0.31×10^6 binding sites per cell unless the affinity of the MAb exceeded 10×10^8 M^{-1}. When at least 10^6 antigenic sites per cell were demonstrable in vitro, MAbs with affinities as low as 0.7×10^8 M^{-1} successfully localized tumours in vivo.

A statistically significant correlation ($r = 0.84$, $p < 0.05$; and $r = 0.81$, $p < 0.05$ for % injected dose/g and localization index, respectively) was found between the sum of the ln of the number of binding sites and of the association constant and the ability of MAbs to localize tumours in vivo (Fig. 2).

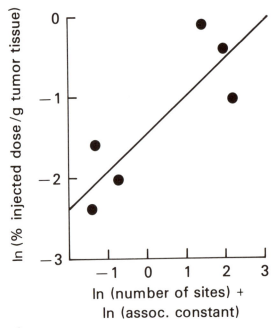

Figure 2.
Correlation between the summed ln of number of binding sites and association constant and the ln of % injected dose/g tumour tissue ($r = 0.84$, $p < 0.05$) established for six anti-melanoma MAbs.

The products of the two in vitro binding parameters ranged between 4.34 and 9.62 for the effective MAbs; those for the inefficient MAbs were between 0.21 and 0.54 (not shown). Although the association constant alone appeared somewhat useful in predicting in vivo localization of MAbs, the correlation was not significant ($r = 0.77$, $p > 0.05$; and $r = 0.72$, $p > 0.05$ for % injected dose/g and localization index, respectively).

DISCUSSION

The iodinated $F(ab')_2$ fragments of the five MAbs that successfully radioimaged human tumour xenografts in nude mice showed significantly higher tumour-to-tissue ratios of radioactivity, higher localization indices and higher specific activities in tumour tissues as compared to the values obtained with the three non-radioimaging MAbs.

Our results strongly suggest that both MAb binding affinity and density of MAb binding sites on tumour cells are important factors in tumour localization. Comparison of anti-melanoma MAbs ME D63 and ME C44, for example, which are directed against the same antigen but to different determinants (17), showed that only the former, with higher binding affinity and number of antigenic sites, clearly radioimaged the tumour xenografts.

For CRC and melanoma tumour grafts with at least 10^6 MAb binding sites per cell, antibodies with affinities as low as 0.7×10^8 M^{-1} successfully localized tumours in vivo. When 3.1×10^5 or less sites per cell were available, affinities of at least 10^9 M^{-I} were required for MAbs to radioimage the tumours. We could clearly demonstrate a significant correlation between either the localization index or the specific activity in tumour tissues (expressed as % injected dose/g tissue) and the product (or sum of the ln) of MAb binding affinity and number of antibody molecules bound (Fig 2). No significant correlation was seen in statistical analyses using either of the two in vitro binding parameters alone.

Anti-melanoma MAbs ME 37-7 and ME 82-11 had binding affinities and antigen densities similar to or greater than those of either of the anti-CRC MAbs, yet radioimaged the tumours less well than the anti-CRC MAbs. This was substantiated by the greater accumulation of specific activities of radioactivity (expressed as % injected dose/g tissue, Table 4) in CRC tumours than in melanomas. It is difficult to explain the differences in MAb localization observed in the two tumour systems. No differences in the vascularity, vascular permeability or tumour blood flow, as reflected by similar non-specific uptake of control MAb by both CRC and melanoma tissue, were detected, nor were differences revealed in the proportion of either necrotic or host inflammatory tissue present in histological preparations. Although the clearance rates of radiolabelled MAbs from CRC tumours between days 2 and 4 did not differ significantly from the rates obtained with melanomas (not shown), further investigations at earlier time points may reveal such differences. Experiments by other in vivo and in vitro have shown both rapid (12) and slow (28,29) clearance of iodinated antibodies from tumour cells.

Shedding of tumour-associated antigens by the target cells did not seem to be of importance for tumour localization by MAbs since tumours were visualized by MAbs directed against shed antigens (CO 2032, ME 37-7, ME D63) as well as by MAbs directed against antigens that are not shed (CO 17-1A, ME 82-11). This observation contrasts with reports by others (11,13) indicating that tumour-associated antigens circulating in vivo may interfere with tumour locaalization by antibodies via the formation of antigen-antibody immune complexes.

Although multiple factors determine the usefulness of radiolabelled MAbs for the localization of malignant disease in cancer patients, our results demonstrate a significant correlation between MAb binding affinity and antigen density on tumour cells and the efficiency of the MAbs to localize tumours in vivo. This suggests that the in vitro binding assays may be an effective means to screen for MAbs with tumour radiolocalization potential.

REFERENCES

1. Colcher D, Zalutsky M, Kaplan W., et al:
   Radiolocalization of human mammary tumours in athymic mice by a monoclonal antibody. Cancer Res 43:736–742, 1983.

2. Pimm M.V., Embleton M.J., Perkins A.C., et al:
   In vivo localization of anti-osteogenic sarcoma 791T monoclonal antibody in osteogenic sarcoma xenografts. Int. J. Cancer 20:20–85, 1982.

3. Mach J.P. Buchegger F., Forni M., et al: Use of radio-labelled monoclonal anti-CEA antibodies for the detection of human carcinoma by external photoscanning and tomoscintigraphy. Immunol Today 2:239–249, 1981.

4. Moshakis V., McIlhinney R.A.J., Raghavan D., et al: Localization of human tumour xenografts after i.v. administration of radiolabelled monoclonal antibodies. Br. J. Cancer 44:91–99, 1981.

5. Salter D., Ballou B., Reilan J., et al:
   Radioimmunodetection of tumours using monoclonal antibodies. In Hybridomas in Cancer Diagnosis and Treatment. Mitchel M.S. and Oettgen H.F. (eds), New York,

NY, Raven Press, 1982, pp 241-244.

6. Hedin A., Wahren B., Hammarstrom S.: Tumour localization of CEA-containing human tumours in nude mice by means of monoclonal anti-CEA antibodies.
Int. J. Cancer 30:547-552, 1982.

7. Shimizu K., Reintgen D., Coleman R.E., et al: In vivo and in vitro binding of iodinated monoclonal antibody against RIN insultimona cells.
Hybridoma 2:26-77, 1983.

8. Khaw B., Strauss H., Cahill S., et al: Sequential imaging of indium-111 labelled monoclonal antibody in human mammary tumours hosted in nude mice.
J. Nucl. Med. 25:592-603, 1984.

9. Herlyn D., Powe J., Alavi A., et al: Radioimmunodetection of human tumour xenografts by monoclonal antibodies.
Cancer Res 43:2731-2735, 1983.

10. Powe J., Pak K.Y., Paik C.H., Steplewski Z., et al: Labelling monoclonal antibodies and $F(ab')_2$ fragments with (^{111}In) indium using cyclic DTPA anhydride and their in vivo behavior in mice bearing human tumour xenografts. Cancer Drug Delivery 1:125-135, 1984.

11. Warenius H., Galfre G., Bleehen N., Milstein C.: Attempting targeting of a monoclonal antibody in a human tumour xenograft system. Eur. J. Cancer Clin. Oncol. 17:1009-1015, 1981.

12. Froese G., Berczi I., Israels L.G.: Tumour cell-antibody interactions - I. In vivo experiments.
Immunology 45:303-312, 1982.

13. Hagen P.L. Halperns S.E. Chen A., et al: Effect of tumour size, carcinoembryonic antigen (CEA) production and

secretion on the distribution of ^{111}In and ^{125}I
monoclonal anti-tumour antibodies (MoAb) in animal models
(abstract). J. Nucl. Med. p. 24:77, 1983.

14. Herlyn M., Steplewski Z., Herlyn D., et al:
Production and characterization of monoclonal antibodies
against human malignant melanoma.
Cancer Invest 1:215-224, 1983.

15. Koprowski H., Steplewski Z., Herlyn D., et al:
Studies of antibodies against human melanoma produced by
somatic cell hybrids. Proc. Natl. Acad. Sci USA
75:3405-3409, 1978.

16. Mithcell K., Ward F., Koprowski H.: DR antigens on
melanoma cells: analysis with monoclonal antibodies.
Human Immunol. 4:15-26, 1982.

17. Herlyn D., Powe J., Ross A.H., et al: Tumour growth
inhibition by IgG2a monoclonal antibodies correlates with
antibody density on tumour cells. J.Immunol., in press.

18. Ross A., Cossu G., Herlyn M., et al: Isolation and
chemical characterization of a melanoma-associated
proteoglycan antigen. Arch. Biochem. Biophys.
225:370-383, 1983.

19. Ross A., Grob P., Bothwell M., et al: Characterization of
nerve growth factor receptor in neural crest tumours using
monoclonal antibodies. Proc. Natl. Acad. Sci. USA, in press.

20. Steplewski Z., Herlyn M., Herlyn D., et al: Reactivity of
monoclonal anti-melanoma antibodies with melanoma cells
freshly isolated from primary and metastatic melanoma.
Eur. J. Immunol. 9:94-96, 1979.

21. Herlyn M., Steplewski Z., Herlyn D., et al: Colorectal
carcinoma specific antigen: Detection by means of

monoclonal antibodies. Proc. Natl. Acad. Sci. USA
76:1438-1442.

22. Blaszczyk M., Pak K., Herlyn M., et al: Characterization
of gastrointestinal tumour-associated carcinoembryonic
antigen-related antigens defined by monoclonal antibodies.
Cancer Res 44:245-253, 1984.

23. Woodbury R.G., Brown J.P. Hellstrom I., et all:
Identification of a cell surface protein in human melanomas
and certain other neoplasms. Proc. Natl. Acad. Sci. USA
77:2183-2187, 1980.

24. Trucco M., Petris, S.: Determination of equilibrium
binding parameters of monoclonal antibodies specific for
cell surface antigens. In Immunological Methods, Lefkovits
I. and Pernis B. (eds), Vol. II. New York, Academic Press,
1981, pp 1-26.

25. Scatchard G.: The attraction of proteins for small
molecules and ions. Ann NY Acad. Sci. 51:660-672, 1949.

26. Ott L.: Inferences related to linear regression and
correlation. In An Introduction to Statistical Methods and
Data Analysis, 2nd edition, Boston, Duxbury Press, 1984,
pp. 280-316.

27. Froese G., Berczi I., Israels L.: Tumour cell-antibody
interactions. II. In vitro studies.
Immunology 45:313-323, 1982.

28. Schlom J., Colcher D., Horan-Hand P., et al: Detection and
enhancement of antigens associated with human mammary
and colon cancer (abstract). Hybridoma 3:58, 1984.

29. Dean C., Hobbs S., Hopkins J., et al: Syngeneic antitumour
antibodies in rats: clearance of cell-bound antibody in
vivo and in vitro. Br. J. Cancer 46:190-197, 1982.

Clinical Application of Numerical Analysis to Radioimmunolocalisation

Green A.J., Begent R.H.J., Searle F. and Bagshawe K.D.

Cancer Research Campaign Laboratories, Department of Medical Oncology, Charing Cross Hospital, London W6 BRF, U.K.

INTRODUCTION

Radioimmunoscintigraphy (RIS) using background subtraction techniques has been reported to be capable of providing images of a number of different tumours in man. Whilst it is reasonably easy to image large deposits of tumour with this technique there is still a need to demonstrate its utility in clinical decision making.

We have investigated the use of RIS in the problem of early localisation of recurrent tumours. In colorectal carcinoma, choriocarcinoma and germ cell tumours the presence of recurrent tumour may be predicted from a rise in serum levels of specific tumour markers (carcinoembryonic antigen (CEA), human chorionic gonodotrophin (hCG) and alphafetoprotein (AFP) respectively). It is clinically important to locate the sites of recurrence as early as possible. This study investigates our previously published analysis method (Green et al, J. Nucl. Med. (1984) 25: 96–100) in these diseases and specifically investigates the method in the early detection of recurrent tumour where the level of serum tumour marker is elevated but the tumour site is not evident on clinical examination.

ANTIBODIES AND PATIENTS

Four antibodies were used for the study:

PK1G (D2)   a goat polyclonal antibody to CEA

11-258-14   a mouse monoclonal antibody to CEA

W14   a mouse monoclonal antibody to HCG

161   a mouse monoclonal antibody to AFP

The antibodies were highly purified, all could be iodinated with ^{131}Iodine (^{131}I) by modified chlormine T methods. Protein doses were between 50 and 200 ug, ^{131}I doses were between 0.5 and 1.5 mCi.

Patients having regular serum marker radioimmunoassay following resection of primary or secondary cancer or chemotherapy were investigated by RIS, x-ray computed tomography (CT), ultrasound (US), or other tests as thought appropriate if serum markers were raised.

SCANNING AND ANALYSIS

All the RIS studies were done using the same technique. Following a negative skin test the appropriate labelled antibody was given intravenously. After 24 hr 0.5 mCi of ^{99m}Technetium (^{99m}Tc) was given as pertechnetate followed after 20 min by 0.5 mCi of ^{99m}Tc labelled Human Serum Albumin. Imaging on a Nuclear Enterprises LFOV gamma camera was started immediately. Images were taken in pairs at 364 KeV for ^{131}I and 140 keV for ^{99m}Tc, at least 250k counts were collected in each. The images were computer smoothed and stored for later analysis by the method of Green et al. Briefly, in this method two regions within the same organ or tissue are selected and the ratio of ^{131}I counts in the two regions is compared with the ratio of ^{99m}Tc counts in the same regions. If neither region is tumour bearing the ratios should not be significantly different. A value (Fx) is computed as the number of standard deviations by which the ratio of counts in the ^{131}I image exceeds the ratio of counts in the ^{99m}Tc image. Computer subtraction images were used as a guide for region drawing.

RESULTS

Figures 1 to 3 show the Fx results obtained in the three diseases. Fig. 1 gives the results for colorectal cancer, fig. 2 for choriocarcinoma and fig. 3 for germ cell tumours.

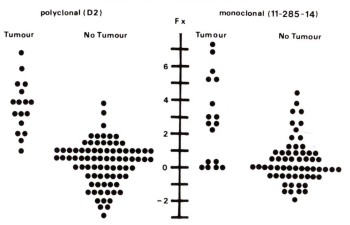

Fig. 1.

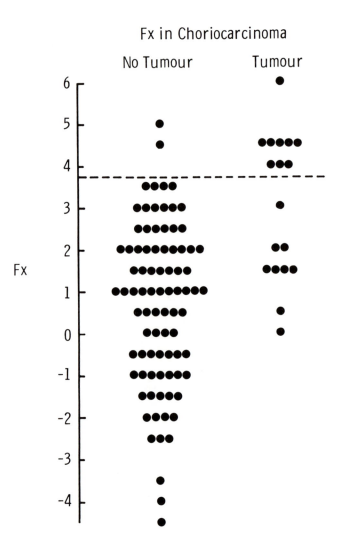

Fig. 2.

161 Antibody to AFP

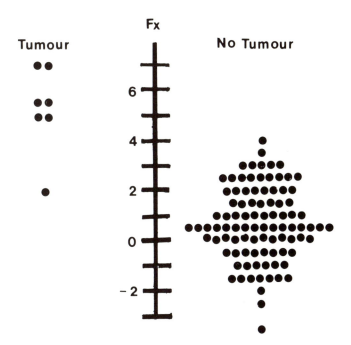

Fig. 3.

Results for confirmed tumour bearing regions are shown to the left of the axis and those in which no tumour was found are shown to the right. In all cases it can be seen that the tumour and non tumour containing regions form different groups. Non parametric statistical analysis of the data for two anti CEA antibodies and the anti hCG antibody show the groups of tumour bearing regions to be significantly different from the non tumour groups at a 5% level. This analysis was not carried out for the smaller group in the germ cell tumours although qualitatively the results appear similar to those in the other diseases.

Non parametric statistical tests of the data for colorectal carcinoma do not show a significant difference between the tumour regions for the two antibodies to CEA and so, in fig. 1, the cluster of Fx values close to zero for the monoclonal antibody are not regarded as significant. The analysis also shows no difference between the non tumour regions for the two antibodies.

It is difficult to quantify the role which RIS played in the diagnosis for many of the patients in this study. RIS was often one in a number of investigations carried out (CT, US etc.) and the results of all the tests were taken into consideration in the final assessment.

Fx values greater than 4 were taken as positive findings and Fx values in the range of 2 to 4 were taken as equivocal.

In an example raised serum AFP and positive RIS using antibody to AFP with negative US and CT was followed by surgical intervention and the removal of a 1 cm tumour after which the serum AFP level returned to normal. In other cases RIS preceeded CT or US scanning and was useful for indicating which regions should be investigated.

These examples were anecdotal and larger patient numbers are needed for a full analysis. However, they do serve to illustrate the potential of RIS.

CONCLUSIONS

We have shown that using antibodies to CEA in colorectal cancer, hCG in choriocarcinoma and AFP in germ cell tumours RIS by the Fx analysis technique is useful in the detection of early recurrent tumour. In some cases RIS appears to be capable of giving information not available from other scanning methods.

Melanoma-Associated Antigens in Human Skin Malignant Melanoma and Benign Nevocytic Tumours

Ranki A.[1], Niemi K.M.[1], Asko-Jeljavaara S[2], Atkinson B.[3], Steplewski Z[3], Herlyn M.[3], Koprowski H.[3]

1. Department of Dermatology, University Central Hospital, University of Helsinki, Finland.
2. IV Department of Surgery, University Central Hospital, University of Helsinki, Finland.
3. The Wistar Institute of Anatomy and Biology, Philadelphia, P.A., U.S.A.

INTRODUCTION

Panels of monoclonal antibodies against human malignant melanoma have been produced by several groups during the past years (for references, see Hybridoma, Vol. 1 (4), 1982). Most of the antibodies, however, have not been sufficiently specific for clinical use. Moreover, the antigenic structures have not withstood routine formalin fixation procedures (1, 2, 3). Such antibodies would, however, be useful in studying the melanoma-associated antigens shared by benign nevocytic tumours and different types and levels of melanoma in order to better understand the antigenic heterogeneity of malignant melanoma. This would give important basic information to be used in applying the monoclonal antibodies for clinical use in tumour imaging studies and therapeutic interventions.

In this study, a panel of eight selected monoclonal anti-melanoma antibodies produced at Wistar Institute were used to characterize the melanoma-associated antigens in fresh biopsies of human skin melanomas and benign nevocytic tumours.

MATERIALS AND METHODS

Monoclonal antibodies. Hybridomas of mouse myeloma cells and splenocytes of mice immunized with human melanoma cell lines, crude membranes of melanoma cells or with a crude melanosome preparation were produced as described previously (1, 4, 5, 6). The antibodies produced were screened by radioimmunoassay and mixed hemadsorption assay for binding to human tumour and normal cell lines (7). As control antibodies, monoclonal antibodies against Concanavalin A lectin (a gift from Dr. P. Ashorn) and monoclonal anti-human milk fat globulin antibody (8) were used.

Characterization of antigens detected. The biochemical analysis of the antigens detected was performed with immunoprecipitation and immunoaffinity chromatography as described is detail elsewhere (9).

Tissue samples. Fresh surgical biopsies of nine primary melanomas and five metastatic melanomas of human skin, altogether 40 nevocytic tumours, three solitary basal cell carcinomas, three seborrheic warts, one lentigo simplex and 2 biopsies of hypermelanotic skin were obtained. In addition, 20 biopsies of normal human skin were taken. All samples were immediatedly frozen in liquid nitrogen and cryostate sections were made.

Immunohistochemistry. Biotin-avidin immunoperoxidase staining was performed as described previously (10) using the Vectastain kit

160

(Vector Laboratories, Burlingame, CA). The sections were fixed with cold acetone or paraformaldehyde. The monoclonal anti-melanoma antibodies were used in 1:20 dilution (optimal dilution). The control antibodies were used in 1:200 dilution.

Routine hematoxylin-eosin staining was made of each biopsy for histopathologic diagnosis.

RESULTS

The antibodies used represented a panel of antibodies ranging from those restricted to react with melanomas only (Group I, Table 1) to those reacting with astrocytomas and other tumours as well (Group IV, Table 1).

Table 1

Characterization of the anti-melanoma antibodies and the respective antigens

Group[a]	Antibodies Included	Antigen detected
I	B1-77-71	Not identified
II	131-2-H6-1, G_1-15-43	proteoglycan
	H_4-18-90, 691-19-19	(260-290 kd)
III	I_1-82-13	75 kd, NGF receptor[b]
IV	9-19-26[c]	not characterized
–	ME-492	protein, 30-60 kd

[a] According to the binding pattern to a variety of human cells and for reference see Herlyn et all., 1982. Comparative study of the binding characteristics of monoclonal antimelanoma antibodies.

161

Hybridoma 1: 403-411.

*b)Ross A.H., Grob P., Bothwell M., Elder D.E., Ernst C.S., Marano N., Christ B.F.D., Slemp C.C., Herlyn M., Atkinson B., and Koprowski H. 1984. Identification of a melanoma-associated antigen as the nerve growth factor receptor. Proc. Natl. Acad. Sci. U.S.A. in press.

c)Antibody of IgM isotype.

In addition, a recently developed antibody against a protein antigen was also included (ME 492). The optimal conditions for immunohistochemical staining of frozen sections was first studied, the most suitable fixative was cold acetone followed by biotin-avidin immunoperoxidase staining.

The irrelevant anti-ConA and anti-HMFG antibodies gave negative staining results on both malignant melanomas and benign nevi. None of the anti-melanoma antibodies reacted with any of the non-melanocytic or non-nevocytic tumours studied. In normal human skin, cells of macrophage morphology scattered in the dermis were stained with the IgM type antibody, Group IV and ME 492 antibodies (Table 2). Some of these cells might have been also mast cells as suggested by their localization and granular pattern. Out of other cells, Group III antibody stained sweat glands. Infiltrating lymphocytes or other structures of the skin were not stained by any of the antibodies. Group II and III antibodies as well as ME 492 antibody stained single cells here and there along the basal layer of the epidermis (Fig. 1). By light microscopy it was not possible to determine whether these cells were of melanocyte or keratinocyte origin. The occurrence of these cells was not related to the amount of pigment and long bits of negatively stained epidermis was usually seen in between.

Table 2

Immunohistochemical reactivity of anti-melanoma antibodies with human nevocytes and melanoma cells in frozen skin samples.

Cell type	Antibodies				
	Group I	Group II	Group III	Group IV	ME 491
Junctional nevocytes	0/3	5/19	0/5	0/13	6/13
Intradermal[a] nevocytes	0/11	17/20	1/13	2/19	7/10
Melanoma[b] cells	1/13	10/14	4/17	8/14	8/8
Basal layer cells in epidermis	0/16	13/26	2/10	0/26	11/19
Normal skin	0/20	0/5	0/5[c]	0/21[d]	0/5[d]

[a] Includes also nevocytes of compound nevi, blue nevi and halo nevi.

[b] Includes both primary and metastatic melanomas, see also Table 3.

[c] Sweat glands stained.

[d] Macrophages stained.

Group I antibody was restricted to melanomas but only one (Clark level IV) melanoma was positive (Fig. 2) and all the metastases were negative. Group II antibodies showed a considerably similar reactivity in all samples and thus the results are given combined.

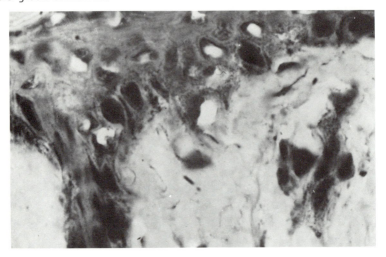

Figure 1.

Normal human skin stained with group III antibody.
Reaction visualized with diaminobenzidine. x 400.

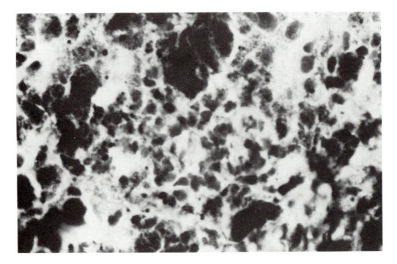

Malignant melanoma of Clark level IV stains with group
I antibody. x 160.
Table 3.

The expression of melanoma-associated antigens of melanoma
tumours of different anatomical levels (Clark's classification).

Stage	Group I	Group II	Group III	Group IV	ME 492
Clark I	0/2	1/2	ND	1/2	1/1
Clark II	0/1	1/1	ND	0/2	ND
Clark III	0/1	2/2	ND	1/2	ND
Clark IV	1/2	3/3	1/1	2/3	2/2
Clark V	0/1	0/1	0/1	0/1	1/1
Metastases	0/5	4/5	0/5	3/5	4/4

These antibodies reacted with most melanomas and melanoma
metastases. The staining pattern in the malignant cells was mostly
cytoplasmic (Fig.3). However, in most benign nevi positive staining
was observed with these antibodies in most of the nevocytes. Here,
the staining pattern was more membranous although no clear-cut
conclusions could be made by light microscopy. In intradermal and
compound nevi, the nevocytes located right below the epidermis or
at lowest parts of the tumour were usually stained. In junctional
nevi, the nests within the epidermis were strongly positive, almost
in a cytoplasmic pattern (Fig. 4). Group III antibody stained less
melanomas than group II antibodies but positive staining was seen
in only one nevus with this antibody. No junctional nevocytes
reacted with this group 111 antibody.

Group IV antibody stained about half of the melanomas (both primary and metastatic, Fig. 5) and reacted with benign nevocytes in only two cases. Again, no junctional nevocytes were stained.

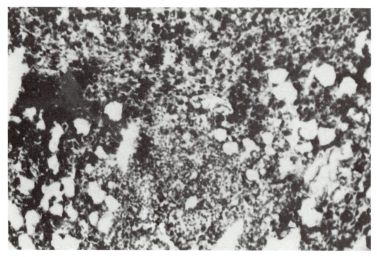

Figure 3.
Malignant melanoma of Clark level IV stained with Group II antibody. x 100.

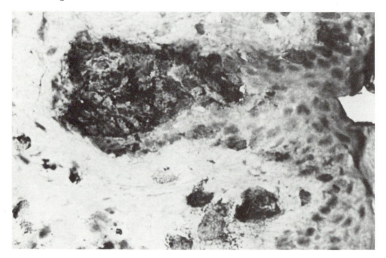

Figure 4.
Nest of nevocytes within the epidermis in a junctional nevus.
Stained with group II antibody. x 400.

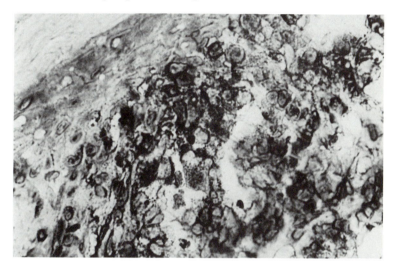

Figure 5.
Malignant melanoma of Clark level I stained with group IV
antibody. x 400.

The antibody produced against melanosome fraction, ME 491,
stained all melanomas, both primary and metastatic, but also
reacted with most benign nevocytes, both junctional (Fig. 6) and
intradermal.

Out of the different types of nevus tumours, no difference in
the staining pattern of halo nevi or blue nevi (Fig. 7) compared to
the other nevi was observed. Melanophages were not stained
except in the blue nevi.

Comparing the reactivity of the malignant melanomas with the
presented antibody panel to the level of tumour invasion (Table 3),

no differences were seen. All melanomas and metastases studied reacted with at least one of the antibodies but none of the tumours reacted with all antibodies.

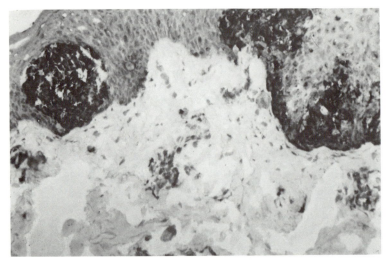

Figure 6

Junctional nevocytes stained with antibody ME 492. x 160

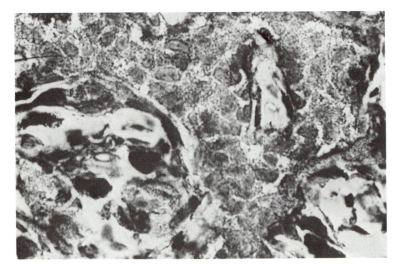

Figure 7

Part of a blue nevus, stained with group II antibody. x 400.

Within the melanoma tumours and the metastases, the majority of the cells usually reacted with the appropriate antibody but small clusters of negative malignant cells could often be seen.

DISCUSSION

The results confirm that melanoma cells show a heterogeneous pattern of antigen expression (11, 12, 13, 14) that can be demonstrated even within the same tumour. No stage-specific antigens could be observed although the possibility that a larger quantity of material would have revealed an antigenic pattern associated with e.g. an aggressive type of melanoma can not be ruled out. A decrease in the expression of melanoma-associated antigens has been reported to occur in the more advanced tumours (14) but this phenomenon could not be seen in our material. As frozen sections were used, our results can be taken to be relevant to the in vivo expression of the melanoma-associated antigens.

The antigenic heterogeneity was not only seen in melanomas but also in the compound and intradermal nevi. In these benign tumours the positively stained cells were mostly those close to the epidermal junction and, on the other hand, those in the deepest parts of the nevi. This may suggest variation in the level of differentiation of the nevocytes.

A striking feature was the strong positive staining pattern in the junctional nevocytes in the nests within the epidermis. Their cytoplasmic type of staining resembled that of the malignant melanoma cells. As most melanomas arising in pre-existing nevi originate in at the epidermal-dermal junction, it is of interest that

169

in about half of the junctional and compound nevi, expression of melanoma-associated antigens can be seen.

The antigenic pattern seen in the different nevi of one individual was variable (data not shown) suggesting rather a cell-line specificity of the antigens than allospecificity. As there were no multiple metastases of a single melanoma in these series, the possible clonality of the malignant cells cannot be commented.

The expression of melanoma-associated antigens in the cells of the basal layer in epidermis has been observed by other investigators, too (12, 13). Our preliminary immunoelectron microscopic studies suggest these cells to be rather keratinocytes than melanocytes or exocytic cells (Dr. R. Caputo and Dr. E. Berti, personal communication). It is noteworthy that Group I and IV antibodies did not stain these cells. The occurrence of the melanoma-associated antigens in these cells could be due to passive absorption of the secreted products of the near-by melanocytes. Another possibility would be that the antigens represent some growth factors for which the basal keratinocytes possess receptors.

The staining pattern seen with the ME 492 antibody recognising a protein antigen, was quite comparable in the frozen samples to the results obtained in fixed tissue samples (6). Some protein antigens will thus offer an opportunity to produce antibodies also applicable to clinical differential diagnostic use.

Our results suggest that for differential diagnostic purposes, a panel of monoclonal anti-melanoma antibodies can be used. There seems to be a tendency within the antibodies that once the antibody recognizes all melanomas it also reacts with most benign nevocytes and vice versa. However, by using a panel of appropriately chosen antibodies one could rule out the "false"

170

patterns.

The heretogeneity of the malignant melanoma cells in their antigenic expression implies that when using the monoclonal anti-melanoma antibodies for clinical purposes, one should not utilize compounds releasing their effect only into the cells to which the antibody binds (e.g. cytotoxic drugs would be carried to a proportion of the tumour cells, only).

REFERENCES

1. Steplewski Z., Herlyn M., Herlyn D., Clark W.H. and Koprowski H. Reactivity of monoclonal anti-melanoma antibodies with melanoma cells freshly isolated from pprimary and metastatic melanoma. Eur. J. Immunol. 9: 94–96 (1979).

2. Yeh M., Hellstrom I., Brown J.P., Warner G.A., Hansen J.A. and Hellstrom K. Cell surface antigens in human melanoma identified by monoclonal antibody. Proc. Natl. Acad. Sci. U.S.A., 76: 2927–2931 (1979).

3. Carrel S., Accolla R.S., Carmagnoler A.L. and Mach J.P. Common human melanoma-associated antigens detected by monoclonal antibodies. Cancer Res. 40: 2523–2528 (1980).

4. Koprowski H., Steplewski Z., Herlyn D. and Herlyn M. Study of antibodies against human melanoma produced by somatic cell hybrids. Proc. Natl. Acad. Sci., U.S.A., 75:3405–3409 (1978).

5. Herlyn M., Steplewski Z., Herlyn D., Clark W.H., Ross A.H., Blaszczyk M., Pak K.Y. and Koprowski H. Production and characterization of monoclonal antibodies against human malignant melanoma. Cancer Invest 127: 127–136 (1983).

6. Atkinson B., Ernst C.S. Christ B.F.D., Herlyn M., Blaszczyk M., Ross A.H., Herlyn D., Stepkewski Z. and Koprowski H. Identification of melanoma-associated antigens using fixed tissue

screening of antibodies. Cancer Res. 44: 2577-2581 (1984).

7. Herlyn M., Stepkewski Z., Herlyn D. and Kooprowski H. Colorectal carcinoma-specific antigens: Detection by means of monoclonal antibodies. Proc. Natl. Acad. Sci. 76: 1439-1442 (1979).

8. Krohn K., Ashorn P., Helle M. and Ashorn R. Heterogeneity of human milk fat globulin antigens, revealed by monoclonal antibodies. Proceedings of Saariselks Symposium 10-11 August 1983.(This volume)

9. Ross A.H., Cossu G., Herlyn M., Bell J.R. Stepkewski Z. and Koprowski H. Isolation and chemical characterization of a melanoma-associated proteoglycan antigen. Arch. Biochem. Biophys. 225: 370-383 (1983).

10. Ranki A., Kianto U., Kanerva L., Tolvanen E. and Johansson E. Immunohistochemical and electron microscopic characterization of the cellular infiltrate in alopecia (areata, totalis and aniversalis). J. Invest. Dermatol. 83: 7-11 (1984).

11. Natali P.G., Viora M., Nicotra M.R., Giacomini P.., Bigotti A. and Ferrone S. Antigenic hetero-geneity of skin tumours of nonmelanocyte origin: Analysis with monoclonal antibodies to tumour-associated antigens and to histocompatibility antigens. JNCI 71: 439 (1983).

12. Hellstrom I, Carrigues H.J., Cabasco L., Mosely G., Brown J. and Hellstrom K.E. Studies of a high molecular weight human melanoma-associated antigen. J. Immunol. 130: 1467-1472 (1983).

13. Sorg C., Bruggen J., Suter L. and Brocker E.B. Monoclonal antibodies against human malignant melanoma Bull Cancer 70: 113-117 (1983).

14. Bruggen J. Brocker E.B., Suter L., Redmann K. and Sorg C. Comparative analysis of melanoma-associated antigens in primary and metastatic tumour tissue. Contr. Oncol. 19: 139-147 (1984)

Binding Characteristics of radioiodinated monoclonal Antibodies to Melanoma Cells in Vitro and in the nude mouse

S. Matzku[1], O. Kotterer[1], W. Tilgen[2], and
J. Brueggen[3]

[1]Institute of Nuclear Medicine, German Cancer Research
Center, Heidelberg
[2]Dermatological Clinic, University of Heidelberg
[3]Department of Experimental Dermatology, University of
Munster, FRG

Monoclonal anti-tumour antibodies are commonly selected by virtue of their exclusive binding to tumour cells in culture and in histological sections. If antibodies are to be used in vivo, additional criteria have to be fulfilled. These centre around the physiology of antigen expression as well as antibody distribution and breakdown. We report on our activities to define such criteria on the basis of experimental test procedures operating on cultured tumour cells and on tumour transplants in the nude mouse. As a by-product of selecting monoclonal antibodies (MAbs) for tumour targeting in vivo, valuable information on the biology of individual antigen-antibody systems was obtained.

Material

Our studies extended on a series of 7 MAbs selected for binding to melanoma cells (Table 1)

Table 1

Origin and characteristics of anti-melanoma MAbs

Designation	Isotype	Antigen	Source
96.5	IgG 2a	p97	(1)
L10	IgG 1	gp95 (=p97)	(2)
M.2.9.4	IgG 2a	glycoprotein?	(3)
M.2.2.4	IgG 1	glycolipid[1]	(3)
H.4-10-58	IgG 1	glycolipid[1]	(3)
M.2.7.6	IgG 1	?	(3)
M.2.10.15	IgG 1	p200	(3)

[1] both MAbs bind the same antigen

The melanoma cell lines used were representative of the three major morphotypes of melanocyte and melanoma cell differentiation (4) inasmuch as SKMel 25 and MelJuSo correspond to the epitheloid type; MeWo to the bipolar type (pigmented); SKMel 28 and MML-I to the polydendritic type.

Test Procedures

Antigen density

Obviously, the number of antibody binding sites is proportional to the number of antigen molecules per cell. This parameter was determined by exposing increasing amounts of

174

tumour cells to excess labelled MAb for 1h at 0°C (Table 2)

Table 2

Antigen density on cultured melanoma cells

Antigenic binding sites $(x10^4)$ per cell[1]

MAb	MML-I	SKMel 25	SKMel 28	MeWo
96.5	34	4	26	0
L10	n.t.	2	16	0
M.2.9.4	16	10	30	12
M.2.7.6	0.5	3.5	3.8	6-8
M.2.10.15	0.6	9	6	13
M.2.2.4	0.1	0	0.6	0.3
H.4-10-58	0.1	0.1	1.3	0.3

[1]0°, 1h, MAb excess

Two types of antigen density variations were observed. One type was relating to the MAbs used, inasmuch as some Mabs (96.5, M.2.9.4, L10) traced an antigen with high density on most of the cell lines, while others (M.2.2.4, H.4-10-58) identified a low density antigen. The other type was characteristic of tumour cell lines showing a specific pattern of antigen expression: The antigen defined by 96.5 and L10 was absent from MeWo but present on the other lines, while the antigens defined by M.2.7.6 and M.2.10.15 were absent from MML-I but present on the other lines.

(Exhaustive) Absorption of labelled MAbs

175

G

This parameter tells us what proportion of a labelled MAb preparation could ultimately bind to the antigen. It depends on the purity of the MAb preparation (e.g. presence of non-specific light chains) and on the alteration of immunoreactivity by radiolabelling. For practical purposes, exhaustive absorption was approximated by 3 cycles of incubating a fixed amount of labelled MAb with the cell line showing highest antigen density (Tab.3.).

Table 3

Absorption of labelled MAbs by tissue cultured cells

MAb	Cell line	% absorbed[1]	Mode of binding indicative of:
96.5	MML-I	59 %	-2
L10	SK Mel 28	42 %	-2
M.2.9.4	SK Mel 28	75 %	internalization
M.2.7.6	MeWo	46 %	internalization
M.2.10.15	MeWo	21 %	internalization
M.2.2.4	SK Mel 28	8 %	shedding
H.4-10-58	SK Mel 28	10 %	shedding

[1] 200000 cpm of MAb per ml were absorbed in three consecutive cycles with 10^6 live cells per ml for 2h at 37^oC, 5% CO_2 cumulative absorption

[2] neither internalization nor shedding

As can be seen, absorption never reached 100%. In combinations involving antigens of low density, absorption was by no means completed within 3 cycles, although a definite decline was observed in most experiments.

Kinetics of MAb binding (in vitro)

After binding to the antigen, the MAb-antigen complex may persist at the cell surface, or it may be modulated by internalization or by shedding (5). These alternatives could be discrimited (although not definitely proven) by following the time course of binding to live cells and to gluteraldehyde-fixed cells at $37^{\circ}C$ and at $0^{\circ}C$. In addition, pH 2.8 treatment after binding could indicate which proportion of the radiolabelled MAb was still accessible at the cell surface.

A steady increase of binding at $37^{\circ}C$ together with a continuous decrease of the portion desorbed by isotonic buffer of pH 2.8 was taken as indication for modulation by internalization. Binding at $0^{\circ}C$ dominating over $37^{\circ}C$ as well as binding to fixed cells dominating over live cells was an indication of antigen shedding (from metabolically active live cells). Table 3 (far right column) summarizes our evidences. This type of experiment explained why repeated absorption may have declined before being exhaustive (MAbs M.2.2.4 and H.2-10-58).

Antibody release after binding

We were interested in the ultimate fate of bound MAb. To this purpose, binding was performed under various conditions (see above) including pH 2.8 treatment. After washing away unbound antibody cells were incubated for another 72h at 0° and $37^{\circ}C$. Supernatants were counted en precipitated with 10% trichloroacetic acid in order to determine the proportion of

177

protein-bound iodine. A representative experiment is shown in Fig.1. It was observed that release was slow in the absence and rapid in the presence of metabolic activity. Released radioactivity was greater than 90% fixed to protein except with live cells kept at 37°C. In this case, only 40–50% was precipitable with TCA. Hence, internalized MAb did not stay permanently with the binding cell.

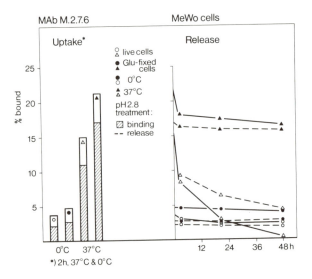

Fig. 1: Release of labelled M.2.7.6 after uptake by MeWo cells

MAb accumulation in vivo

Binding of labelled MAbs to solid melanoma tissue in the nude mouse was followed by comparing the distribution of a relevant MAb and an irrelevant MAb of the same isotype in a paired-label assay (6). Specificity indices (i.e. SI = (MAb in tumour/MAb in normal tissue) / (control Ig in tumour/control Ig in normal tissue)) obtained by this method are presented in Table 4.

Table 4

Specificity indices: MAb accumulation in vivo followed by paired-label experiments

MAb	Tumour	SI(tumour/blood)[1]	SI(tumour/muscle)
M.2.9.4	MeWo	7.7	11.2
M.2.7.6	MML-I	5.5	5.1
M.2.7.6	MeWo	5.5	4.8
M.2.10.15	MeWo	7.4	6.5
H.4-10-58	MeWo	1.2	1.3
M.2.2.4	MML-I	0.9	1.2
M.2.2.4	MeWo	1.0	1.2

[1] Definition of SI in the text. Dissection of tumour bearing nude mide 2 days after application of labelled MAb.

It is understood that SIs around 1 indicate a non-specific distribution. We observed that antigen densities (Table 2) were mostly, but not always mirrored by SIs (see e.g. M.2.7.6 in MML-I

179

tumours). Divergence may be caused by phenotypic shifts from one microenvironment to another. Furthermore, it became obvious that parameters suggestive of antigen shedding gave a reliable prognosis of bad MAb accumulation in vivo (see M.2.2.4 and H.4-10-58). This is at variance with findings in the CEA system (7).Scintigraphic evidence followed closely the picture emerging from SI analysis, i.e. a high SI went together with a good contrast in scintigraphy. This is illustrated with M.2.7.6 (Fig.2.).

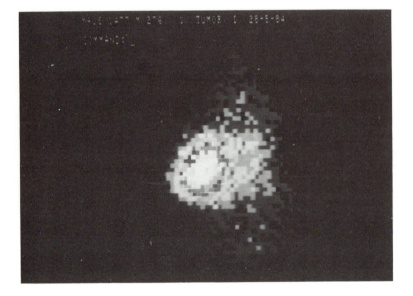

Fig. 2: Scintigraphy of SK Mel 28 transplant in a nude mouse. One day 6 after application of 80 uCi ^{131}I-M.2.7.6, activity was concentrated within the tumour area (head of mouse on top).

If we consider the fact that antibodies against p97 (=gp95) have already been used for immunoscintigraphy, our study elaborated two MAbs as good candidates for in vivo application, namely M.2.7.6 and M.2.10.15. Mab2.9.4 is handicapped by severe cross-expression of the antigen on normal tissue (J.Brueggen & E. Broecker, personal communication), while M.2.2.4 and H.4-10-58 identify an antigen with a clearly unsuitable spectrum of properties.

Conclusion

When evaluating the suitability of a panel of anti-melanoma MAbs for application to the patient, it was found that in most instances antigen density and maximal absorption of labelled antibody correlated with specificity indices of accumlation in vivo. This was also the case when internalization of the antigen-MAb complex was observed. In situations suggestive of antigen shedding, low SIs were obtained. In all combinations tested, high specificity indices were accompanied by good contrast in scintigraphy and vice versa. Two of the MAbs studied might be useful in clinical application, namely M.2.7.6 and M.2.10.15.

Acknowledgement

This work was supported by the Deutsche Forschungsgemeinschaft (SFB 136).

References

1) Brown, J.P., Wright, P.W., Hart, C.E., Woodbury, R.G., Hellstroem, K.E., Hellstroem, I, J. Biol. Chem. 255, 191, 1980.

2) Dippold, W.G., Lloyd, K.O., Li, L.T., Ikeda, H., Oettgen, H.F., Old, L.J., Proc. Natl. Acad. Sci. USA 77, 6114, 1980

3) Suter, L., Broecker, E.B., Brueggen, J., Ruiter, D.J., Sorg, C., Cancer Immunol. Immunother.16, 53, 1983

4) Houghton, A.N., Eisinger, M., Albino, A.P., Cairncross, J.G., Old, L.J., J. Exp. Med. 156, 1755, 1982

5) Chatenoud, L., Bach J.F., Immunlogy today 5, 20, 1984

6) Pressman, D., Day, E.D., Blau, M., Cancer Res. 17, 845, 1957

7) Mach, J.P., Carrel, S., Forni, M., Ritschard, J., Donath, A., Alberto, P., N.Engl. J. Med. 303, 5, 1980

Human Melanoma Associated Antigens recognized by Monoclonal Antibodies

Pullano T.G.[1], Tjujisaki M.[1], Temponi M.[1], Puppo F., Matsui M.[1], Natali P.G.[2] and Ferrone S.[1]

1. Department of Microbiology and Immunology, New York Medical College, Valhalla, New York 10595.
2. Immunlogy Laboratory, Regina Elena Cancer Institute, 00161 Rome, Italy.

INTRODUCTION

Hybridoma technology has been successfully applied by several investigators to develop monoclonal antibodies to human melanoma associated antigens (MAA), i.e. antigens expressed by melanoma cells but not detectable in resting melanocytes (for review, see 1,2,3,4). The high degree of specificity of these reagents has sparked interest in the application of immunological approaches to the diagnosis and treatment of melanoma. Studies performed along these lines have already provided information which could not be obtained with conventional antisera or have rekindled interest in approaches which had been met with limited, if any, success in the past. Thus analysis of surgically removed lesions has identified antigenic profiles characteristic of melanoma cells (5). Furthermore antigenic heterogeneity has been identified among histopathologically indistinguishable lesions taken from different patients, from separate lesions from the same patient, and even within different areas of individual lesions (6). In in-vivo studies monoclonal antibodies have been utilized in radioimaging techniques to visualize metastatic lesions in patients with melanoma (7,8,9,10). In the immunotherapy area monoclonal antibodies conjugated to toxins have been shown to selectively destroy melanoma cells in vitro (11,12,13) and to suppress the growth of transplanted melanoma in nude mice (11,14). A preliminary study with a limited number of patients indicates that anti-MAA monoclonal antibodies labelled with ^{131}I may be a useful tool in immunotherapy of melanoma (8). Such information suggests that immunological parameters may provide new criteria for assessing controversial diagnosis of melanoma and for classifying melanoma lesions. Additionally, the availability of a large panel of anti-MAA monoclonal antibodies will enhance the dissection of antigenic heterogeneity of melanoma cells and will improve the sensitivity of methods to detect melanoma lesions.

In this chapter we will briefly describe the characteristics of a high molecular weight-melanoma associated antigen (HMA-MAA) which has been utilized by participants to this meeting as a marker to radioimage lesions in patients with melanoma thus providing the back ground as to why this antigen was selected for radioimaging studies. Furthermore we will describe an approach to broaden the specificity of anti-MAA monoclonal antibodies.

CHARACTERISTICS OF THE HIGH MOLECULAR WEIGHT-MELANOMA ASSOCIATED ANTIGEN.

The HMA-MAA consists of two non-covalently associated glycopolypeptides: one has an apparent molecular weight of 280K; the other one is composed of a heterogeneous array of glycopolypeptides with molecular weights ranging from 700K to about 300 K (15,16,17). Biosynthetic studies have shown a precursor-product relationship between the 280 K molecular weight component and the larger molecular weight component (16,18). This model is supported by the similarity in composition of peptide maps generated by digesting the two subunits of the HMW-MAA with proteolytic enzymes (17) and by the detection of only one component when the HMW-MAA is purified from melanoma cells incubated with tunicamycin, an inhibitor of N-linked glycosylation (19).

Testing of a large variety of cell lines in long term culture and of a large number of surgically removed normal and malignant tissues has shown that the HMW-MAA has a restricted tissue distribution, since it is expressed only by primary and metastatic melanomas, by nevi, and by less than 50 % of skin carcinomas (20).

Like other types of tumour associated antigens, the HMW-MAA is heterogeneous among lesions isolated from different patients, among autologus lesions isolated from a patient with melanoma and among cells within a lesion (6,21). The extent of heterogeneity of the HMW-MAA is markedly lower than that of other MAAs we have identified with monoclonal antibodies (6). Representative examples are shown in Figure 1.

The level of the HMW-MAA in surgically removed lesions does not correlate with their primary or metastatic nature, with their melanogenic potential and/or with their histopathological characteristics. On the other hand studies in progress suggest that the percentage of tumour cells stained by anti-HMA-MAA and anti-HLA monoclonal antibodies in metastic lesions display some relationship to the degree of malignancy of melanoma (22).

The density of each antigenic determinant recognized by the anti-HMW-MAA monoclonal antibodies (MoAb) 149.55, 225, 28S and

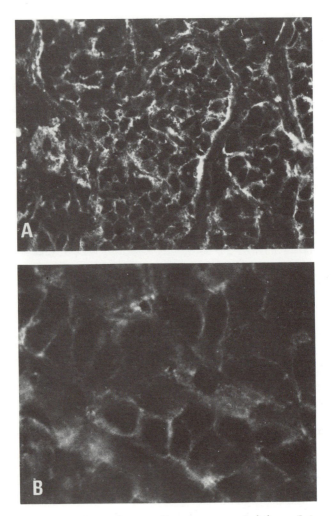

Figure 1a. Indirect immunofluorescence staining of 4u acetone fixed cryostat sections of melanoma metastases with the moAb 225.285 to HMW-MAA (15) (panel A), and with the MoAb 345.134S to 115K MAA (40) (panel B). The HMW-MAA has a relatively homogeneous distribution within a lesion, while the remaining antigens (shown in panel B and in Figures 1b and 1c) have a heterogeneous expression. (A: x650; B: x 1000).

186

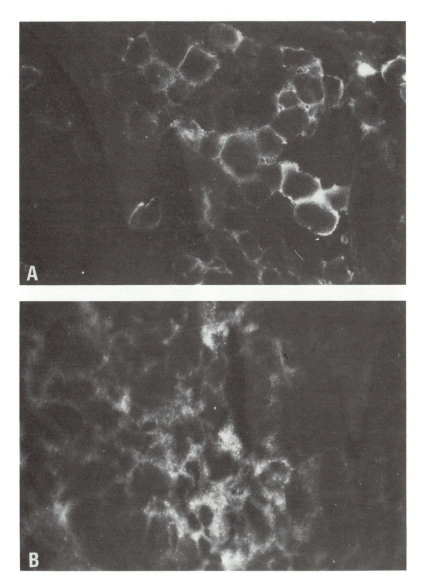

Figure 1b. Indirect immunofluorescence staining performed as in figure 1a, using moAb 376.96 to 100K MAA (41) (panel A), and MoAb 140.240 to 87K MAA (42) (panel B) (x650).

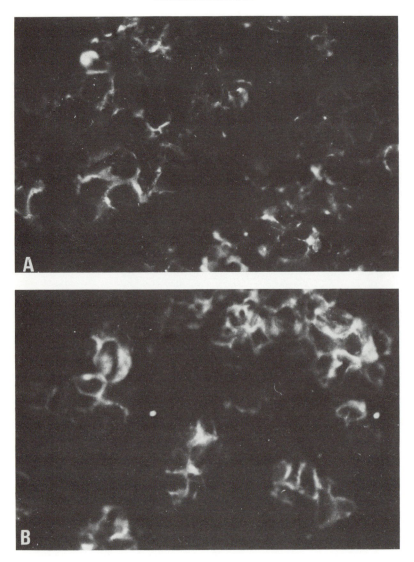

Figure 1c. Indirect immunofluorescence staining performed as in figure 1a, using MoAb M111 elicited with cutaneous melanocytes (43) (panel A) and MoAb A12 to common acute lymphoblastic leukemia antigen (44) (panel B) (x650).

HUMAN MELANOMA ASSOCIATION ANTIGENS

Structural profile and distribution on cell lines in long term culture of
antigens recognized by monoclonal antibodies elicited with IFN-γ treated
cultured melanoma cells Colo 38 +

MoAbs	Molecular Profile	Melanoma cell lines (+)	Melanoma cell lines (-)	Lymphoid cell lines B	Lymphoid cell lines T	Ovary Carcinoma cell lines	Breast Carcinoma line T47D	Hepatocellular carcinoma line PLC
		(+)	(-)	(-)	(-)	(-)	(-)	(-)
VF1-TP36.1 VF1-TP36.2 VF1-TP36.4	118 Kd 95 28 26	Colo 38 WM165-1 WM266-4	DX-2 DX-3 WM35 WM164 WM239A WM115	LG-2 Daudi	JM CCRF-HSB2 Molt-4	SK-OV-4 SK-OV-6 SW626		
		(+)	(-)	(-)		(-)		
VF4-TP170	"	Colo 38 WM164 WM165 WM266-4	DX-2 WM115	LG-2	ND#	SK-OV-4	ND	ND
		(+)		(-)	(-)	(-)	(+)	(+)
VF1-TP53.3	45Kd 42	Colo 38		LG-2 Daudi	JM CCRF-HSB Molt-4	SK-OV-4	(+)	(+)
		(+)	(-)	(-)	(-)	(+)	(+)	(+)
VF1-TP54.9	23.Kd 22.Kd	Colo 38	DX-2	LG-2	Molt-4	SK-OV-4	(+)	(+)
		(+)		(-)	(-)	(+)	(-)	
VF1-TP23	45Kd	Colo 38		LG-2 Daudi	JM CCRF-HSB2 Molt-4	SK-OV-4	(-)	ND
		(+)		(-)	(-)	(+)	(-)	
VF1-TP1	41Kd	Colo 38		LG-2 Daudi	Molt-4 JM CCRF-HSB2	SK-OV-4	(-)	ND
		(+)		(-)	(-)	(-)	(-)	
VF4-TP104	186Kd	Colo 38		LG-2	Molt-4	SK-OV-4	(-)	ND
		(+)		(-)	(-)	(-)	(-)	
VF4-TP112	106Kd 72Kd	Colo 38		LG-2	Molt-4	SK-OV-4	(-)	ND
		(+)		(-)	(-)	(-)	(+)	
VF4-TP159	244Kd 97Kd	Colo 38		LG-2	Molt-4	SK-OV-4	(+)	ND
		(+)		(-)	(-)	(-)	(-)	
CL203.4 CL207.14	100Kd	Colo 38 SK Mel 37		LG-2	Molt-4	SK-OV-4	(-)	ND

The enzyme linked immunosorbent assay (ELISA) was performed in a 96 well, U bottomed plates (Falcon 3911, Becton Dickinson Labware, Oxnard, CA) precoated with phosphate buffered saline, pH 7.0 containing 0.5% non-fat dry milk (DM/PBS). Target cells (1x10⁴) were incubated with 100 μls of antibody solution diluted with DM/PBS, for 60 minutes at 4°C. Following three washings with DM/PBS cells were incubated with 100 μls of an appropriate dilution of horse radish peroxidase conjugated anti-mouse Ig xenoantibodies. At the end of a 60-minute incubation, cells were washed four times and incubated with a freshly prepared substrate solution containing 0.05% o-phenylenediamine and 0.0075% hydrogen peroxide in McIlvain's buffer, pH 6. After a 30 minute incubation at room temperature, absorbance of each test well was read at 405 nm on a Titertek Multiscan plate reader (Flow Laboratories, Inc., McLean, VA). Positive and negative controls were performed utilizing anti-Class I HLA monoclonal antibodies and murine immunoglobulins, respectively. Results were considered positive when the absorbance was at least twice the background values obtained with monoclonal antibodies to unrelated antigens.

Not determined

763.74T on cultured melanoma cells Colo 38 is higher than 2×10^6 sites per cell, as determined by the amount of radiolabelled monoclonal antibody bound by cultured melanoma cells under saturating conditions (22). The incubation of Colo 38 cells with more than one monoclonal antibody to the HMW-MAA has an additive effect suggesting that the number of antigen-antibody interactions on melanoma cell membranes in vivo may be increased by injecting mixtures of monoclonal antibodies to distinct determinants of the HMW-MAA (22).

The HMW-MAA is not susceptible to antibody mediated modulation, since cultured melanoma cells incubated with varying amounts of monoclonal antibodies to a determinant of the HMW-MAA do not change in their ability to bind monoclonal antibodies to other determinants of the HMW-MAA (22). Modulation of the HMW-MAA does not occur even when cultured melanoma cells are incubated with monoclonal antibodies to the HMW-MAA and with anti-mouse Ig antibodies. Furthermore incubation of cultured melanoma cells with monoclonal antibodies to the HMW-MAA does not affect its shedding.

The HMW-MAA has not been detected in normal tissues except for clusters of Malpighian cells in epidermis and hair bulbs (5,20), a conclusion which has been confirmed also by the distribution of radiolabelled anti-HMW-MAA monoclonal antibodies in patients with melanoma and with malignant diseases other than melanoma (9,10). However the HMW-MAA is present in small amount in serum of normal donors (23): the serum HMW-MAA is likely to be derived (shed) from proliferating melanocytes, since this antigen is not detectable on resting melanocytes but is expressed by proliferating melanocytes in culture (24). The level of the HMW-MAA tends to increase in patients with melanoma and the extent of the increase is related to the spreading of the disease (23). Whether a high level of HMW-MAA is serum may have an effect on the biodistribution of anti-HMW-MAA monoclonal antibodies injected into patients with melanoma is not known at present.

DEVELOPMENT OF MONOCLONAL ANTIBODIES TO HUMAN MELANOMA ASSOCIATED ANTIGENS USING IFN-y TREATED MELANOMA CELLS AS IMMUNOGENS.

The range of specificity of murine monoclonal antibodies elicited against cultured human melanoma cells appears to be narrow, although a variety of melanoma cell lines have been used as immunogens and several immunization schedules have been applied. This has resulted in the identification of only a limited number of MAAs. For instance, a single type of HMW-MAA has been identified in five laboratories (15,16,25,26,27). A 95-97 kilodalton MAA has been identified by both Hellstrom (28) and Old (29) and their associates. A cytoplasmic MAA described by Reisfeld and associates (30) and his group (15,31) was found to have a similar structural profile. These results are likely to reflect the immunodominance of particular antigenic molecules, since a wide variety of MAAs have been described using sera from patients with melanoma and antisera from rabbits immunized with human MAAs (for review see 32,33,34,35).

Since a larger panel of monoclonal antibodies to MAA may serve in characterization of melanoma antigenic profiles and in improvement of immunodiagnostic and immunotherapeutic approaches, we have attempted to broaden the specificity of anti-MAA monoclonal antibodies by taking advantage of the dramatic changes in the antigenic profile of melanoma cells induced by treatment with IFN-y. The latter has been shown to reduce the expression of the HMW-MAA, of the 115K MAA recognized by the MoAb 345.134S, and of the 100K MAA recognized by the MoAb 376.96 (36), but to increase the expression of Class I HLA antigens (37), of HLA-DR antigens and of HLA-DQ antigens (38). Increase in the levels of surface HLA anttigens may cause changes in the manner of presentation of other cellular antigens to the mouse immune system. Furthermore, reduction of the levels of immunodiminant cell surface MAAs caused by IFN-y may be associated with an increased immunogenicity of other types of MAAs.

Hybridomas have been constructed utilizing splenocytes from mice immunized with IFN-y treated mleanoma cells, Colo 38. Serological and immunochemical analysis of the specificity of the monoclonal antibodies secreted by the hybridomas has identified some antibodies with a specificity different from that of monoclonal antibodies elicited with untreated mleanoma cells. Representative results are summarized in tables 1 and 2 and in figure 2. The salient observations are as follows:

1. The MoAbs VF1-TP36.1 and ·VF4-TP170 recognize an antigen which consists of 4 subunits with the apparent molecular weights of 118,95,28 and 26 kilodaltons. The antigen is expressed by melanoma cells, but has not been detected on cultured melanocytes, on cultured B and T lymphoid cells, or on cultured breast, hepatocellular and ovary carcinoma cells. The expression of this antigen is not affected by treating cultured melanocytes and melanoma cells Colo 38 with recombinant IFN-y. It is of interest that the MoAbs VF1-TP36.1 and VF4-TP170 display differential reactivity with the various melanoma cell lines tested suggesting that the corresponding determinants may be polymorphic.

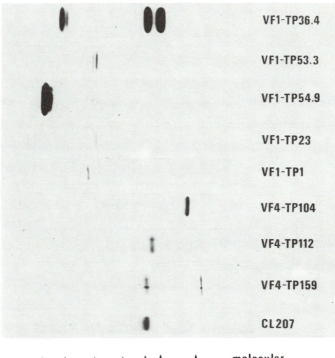

		VF1-TP36.4
		VF1-TP53.3
		VF1-TP54.9
		VF1-TP23
		VF1-TP1
		VF4-TP104
		VF4-TP112
		VF4-TP159
		CL207

molecular weight standards (kilodaltons)

14—22 -31 -45 -66 -93 -116 -200

Figure 2.

Molecular profile of antigens recognized by monoclonal antibodies raised against IFN-y treated melanoma cells Colo 38. The antigens were immunoprecipitated from IFn-y treated Colo 38 cells by antibody CL207 and from untreated Colo 38 cells by the VF1- and VF4- antibodies.

Cell surface antigens on viable Colo 38 cells were radiolabelled with ^{125}I by lactoperoxidase catalyzed iodination (46). Cells were subsequently lysed with 0.5% Triton X-100 in phosphate buffered saline. Lysate was cleared of debris by centrifugation at 100,000 xg and used for indirect immunoprecipitation using Protein A-Sepharose 4B preloaded with

193

rabbit anti-mouse Ig as solid phase absorbant. Immunoprecipitated antigens were denatured in sample buffer and resolved by SDS-PAGE on 3-15% polyacrylamide gradient gels as described by Laemmli (47). After electrophoresis, gels were fixed in 20% methanol, 10% acetic acid in distilled H_2O for 1 hour prior to drying. Autoradiography was performed by exposing dried gels to Kodak X-OMAt X-AR or X-RP film at $-70^{\circ}C$ for 7 to 14 days. Molecular weight standards, radioiodinated by the chloramine T method (48), were myosin (200,000 daltons), B-galactosidase (116,250), phosphorylase B (92,500), bovine serum albumin (66,200), ovalbumin (45,000), carbonic anhydrase (31,000), soybean trypsin inhibitor (21,500), and lysozyme (14,400).

TABLE 2.

Reactivitiy of monoclonal antibodies generated against IFN-y treated melanoma cell line Colo 38, with control and IFN-y treated Colo 38 cells and cultured melanocytes 1168.#

	Colo 38		melanocytes 1168	
	untreated	IFN-y	untreated	IFN-y
VFI-TP23	70*	70	<10	<10
VFI-TP36.4	50	40	<10	<10
VFI-TP54.9	90	80	80	60
CL 203.4	30	70	20	40

Cells were incubated for 72 hours in the presence of IFN-y at a concentration of 500 units/ml prior to testing in the mixed hemagglutination assay (45).

* Data is expressed as percent of cells displaying hemagglutination.

2. The MoAb VF1-TP54.9 recognizes a low molecular weight antigen which is expressed by some of the cultured melanoma cell lines tested, by cultured melanocytes and by the various types of carcinoma cell lines tested. This antigen does not appear to be susceptible to modulation by recombinant IFN-y.

3. The MoAbs VF4-TP104, VF4-TP112 and VF4-TP159 recognize antigens with molecular weights higher than 150 K. These These antigens are expressed by melanoma cells but have not been detected on the lymphoid and carcinoma cell lines tested.

4. The MoAbs CL203 and CL207 recognize a glycoprotein with the apparent molecular weight of 100 K which is expressed on surgically removed melanoma lesions but is not detectable in nevi (39). The antigen is expressed by a small percentage of melanocytes in culture. The level of the antigen is markedly increased on cultured melanoma cells Colo 38 incubated with IFN-y.

CONCLUSIONS

The results we have summarized indicate that through the use of monoclonal antibodies, MAAs have been identified which meet the criteria to be used as markers for radioimaging. Results which are presented by Dr. Buraggi in this meeting indicate that injection of radiolabelled anti-HMW-MAA monoclonal antibodies into patients with melanoma has resulted in the specific accumulation of radioactivity in metastatic lesions.

Furthermore the data we have summarized indicates that the specificity of anti-MAA monoclonal antibodies may be broadened by manipulating the immunogen. The approach we have utilized has taken advantage of the antigenic changes induced by IFN-y. This broadening the specificity of the antibodies may result from the increase in the expression of MAAs which are poorly expressed on untreated cells and from changes in the immunogenicity of antigens associated with the reduced expression of immunodominant MAAs.

REFERENCES

1. Reisfeld R.A., Ferron S. (eds) Melanoma antigens and antibodies. 1982. Plenum Press. New York, London.

2. Steplewski Z. (ed.) Antigens of human melanoma as defined by monoclonal antibodies. Hybridoma 1982; 1:379.

3. Lloyd K.O. Human tumour antigens; Detection and characterization with monoclonal antibodies. In; Herbermann R. ed. Basic and Clinical Tumour Immunology. The Netherlands, Nijhoff, The Hague, 159;214, 1983.

4. Natali P.G., Aguzzi A., Veglia F., Imai K., Burlage R.S., Giacomini P., Ferrone S. The impact of monoclonal antibodies on the study of human malignant melanoma. J. Cutan. Pathol. 10;514-528, 1983.

5. Natali P.G., Bigotti A., Cavaliere R., Nicotra M.R. and Ferrone S. Phenotyping of lesions of melanocyte origin with monoclonal antibodies to melanoma-associated antigens and to HLA antigens. J. Natl. Cancer Inst. 73;13-24, 1984.

6. Natali P.G., Cavaliere R., Bigotti A., Nicotra ME., Russo C., Ng A.G., Giacomini P. and Ferrone, S. Antigenic heterogeneity of surgically removed primary and autologous metastatic human melanoma lesions. J. Immunol. 130;1462-1466, 1983.

7. Larson S.M., Brown J.P., Wright P.W., Carrasquillo J.A., Hellstrom I. and Hellstrom K.E. Imaging of melanoma with ^{131}I labelled monoclonal antibodies. J. Nucl. Med., 24:123:129, 1982.

8. Larson S.M. Carrasquillo J.A., Krohn K.A., Brown J.P.,

McGuffin R.W., Ferens J.M., Graham M.M., Hill L.D., Beumier P.L., Hellstrom K.E. and Hellstrom I. Localization of ^{131}I-labelled p97-specific Fab$_2$ fragments in human melanoma as a basis for radiotherapy. J. Clin. Invest., 72;2101-2114, 1983.

9. Buraggi G.L., Callegaro L., Mariani G., Turrin A., Cascinelli N., Attili A., Bombardieri E., Terno G., Plassio G., Dovis M., Mazzuca N., Natali P.G., Scasselati G., Rosa U. and Ferron S. Imaging with ^{131}I-labelled monoclonal antibodies to a high molecular weight-melanoma associated antigen in patients with melanoma; efficacy of whole Ig and its Fab$_2$ fragments. Submitted 1984.

10. Buraggi G.L., Callegaro L., Turrin A., Cascinelli N., Attili A., Emanuelli H., Gasparini M., Deleide G., Plassio G., Dovis M., Mariani G., Natali P.G., Scassellati G., Rosa U. and Ferrone S. Immunoscintigraphy with ^{123}I, ^{99}Tc and ^{111}In-labelled F(ab)$_2$ fragments of monoclonal antibodies to human high molecular weight-melanoma associated antigen (HMW-MAA). Submitted 1984.

11. Bumol T.F., Wang Q.C., Reisfeld R.A., and Kaplan N.O. Monoclonal antibody and an antibody-toxin conjugate to a cell surface proteoglycan of melanoma cells suppress in vivo tumour growth. Proc. Natl. Acad. Sci. USA 80;529-533, 1983.

12. Casellas P., Brown J.P., Gros O., Gros P., Hellstrom I., Jansen F.K., Poncelet P., Roncucci R., Vidal H. and Hellstrom K.E. Human melanoma cells can be killed in vitro by an immunotoxin specific for melanoma-associated antigen P97. Int. J. Cancer 30;437-443, 1982.

13. Imai K., Nakanishi T., Noguchi T., Yachi S. and Ferrone S. Selective in vitro toxicity of purothionin conjugated to the monoclonal antibody 225,28S to a human high-molecular-weight melanoma associated antigen. Immunother. 15;206-209, 1983.

14. Matsui J., Nakanishi T., Noguchi T., Mai K. and Ferrone S. Suppression of human melanoma growth in nude mice injected with the anti high molecular weight-melanoma associated antigen (HMW-MAA) monoclonal antibody (MoAb) 225.28S conjugated to purothionin. Submitted 1984.

15. Wilson B.S., Iami K., Natali P.G. and Ferrone S. Distribution and molecular characterization of cell-surface and a cytoplasmic antigen detectable in human melanoma cells with monoclonal antibodies. Int. J. Cancer 28;293-300, 1981.

16. Bumol T.F. and Reisfeld R.A. Unique glycoprotein-proteoglycan complex defined by monoclonal antibody on human melanoma cells. Proc. Natl. Acad. Sci. USA 9;1245-1249, 1982.

17. Wilson B.S., Ruberto G. and Ferrone S. Immunochemical characterization of a human high molecular weight melanoma-associated antigen identified with monoclonal antibodies. Cancer Immunol. Immunother. 14;196-201, 1983.

18. Kantor R.R.S., Ng A.K., Giacomini P., Albino A.P. and Ferrone S. Biosynthesis of four human melanoma-associated antigens. Fed. Proc. 42;565, 1983.

19. Gold A.M., Kantor R.S., Giacomini P., Ng A.K., Steinbach G. and Ferrone S. Heterogeneity and topography of determinants recognized by monoclonal antibodies on a human high molecular-weight-melanoma associated antigen. Recent Adv. in Analytical Methodology in the Life Sciences. Proc. 8th U.S. Food & Drug Admin. Science Symposium, pp. 316-332, 1983.

20. Natali P.G., Imai K., Wilson B.S., Bigotti A., Cavaliere R., Pellegrino M.A. and Ferrone S. Structural properties and tissue distribution of the antigen recognized by the monoclonal antibody 653.40S to human melanoma cells. J. Natl. Cancer Inst. 67;591-601,

1981.

21. Natali P.G., Bigotti A., Cavaliere R., Liao K., Taniguchi M., Matsui M. and Ferrone S. Melanoma associated antigens and HLA antigens autologous lesions surgically removed from patients with melanoma. Submitted, 1984.

22. Ferrone S., Giacomini P., Natali P.G., Ruiter D., Buraggi G., Callegaro L. and Rosa U. A ˙human high molecular weight-melanoma-associated antigen (HMW-MAA) defined by monoclonal antibodies: A useful marker to radioimage tumour lesions in patients with melanoma. In* Proc. 1st Internat'l Symp. on Neutron Capture Therapy. Brookhaven National Laboratory, pp. 174-183, 1983.

23. Giacomini P., Veglia F., Cordiali Fei P., Rehle T., Natali P.G. and Ferrone S. Level of membrane-bound high-molecular-weight-melanoma-associated antigen and a cytoplasmic melanoma-associated antigen in surgically removed tissues and sera from patients with melanoma. Cancer Res. 44:1281-1287, 1984.

24. Lloyd K.O., Albino A. and Houghton A. Analysis of hybridoma-exchange antibodies. Hybridoma, 1;461-463, 1982.

25. Carrel S., Accolla R.S., Carmagnola A., Mach J.P. Common human melanoma-associated antigens(s) detected by monoclonal antibodies. Cancer Res. 40:2523-2528, 1980.

26. Hellstrom I., Carrigues H.J., Cabasco L., Mosley G.G., Brown J.P. and Hellstrom K.E. Studies of a high molecular weight human melanoma-associated antigen. J. Immunol. 130;1367-1472, 1983.

27. Ross A.H., Cossu G., Herlyn M. Bell J.R., Steplewski Z., Koprowski H. Isolation and chemical characterization of a melanoma-associated proteoglycan antigen. Arch. Biochem.

Biophys. 225:370–383, 1983.

28. Brown J.P., Woddbury R.G., Hart C.E., Hellstrom I., Hellstrom K.E. Quantitative analysis of melanoma associated antigen p97 in normal and neoplastic tissues. Proc. Natl. Acad. Sci. USA, 78539–543, 1981.

29. Dippold W.G., Lloyd K.O., Li L.T.C., Ikeda H., Oettgen H.F. and Old L.J. Cell surface antigens of human malignant melanoma: definition of six antigenic systems with mouse monoclonal antibodies. Proc. Natl. Acad. Sci. USA, 77:6114–6118, 1980.

30. Bumol T.F., Chee D.O. and Reisfeld R.A. Immunochemical and biosynthetic analysis of monoclonal antibody-defined melanoma-associated antigen. Hybridoma, 1:283–2292, 1982.

31. Natali P.G., Wilson B.S., Imai K., Bigotti A. and Ferrone S. Tissue distribution, molecular profile and shedding of a cytoplasmic antigen identified by the monoclonal antibody 465.12S to human melanoma cells. Cancer Res. 42:583–589, 1982.

32. Ferrone S. and Pellegrino M.A. Serological detection of human melanoma associated antigens. In: Immunodiagnosis; (R.B. Herberman and R. McIntire, eds.) Marcel-Dekker, New York, p. 588–632, 1979.

33. Brown J.M. and Rosenberg S.A. In "Immunological Approaches to Cancer Therapeutics: E. Mihich, ed.), 1982, J. Wiley, and Sons, Inc.

34. Heaney-Kieras J. and Bystryn J.C. Identification and purification of a M_r 75,000 cell surface human melanoma-associated antigen. Cancer Res. 42:2310–2316, 1982.

35. Mattes M.J., Jolis M., Thompson T.M., Old L.J. and Lloyd K.O. A pigmentation-associated, differentiation antigen of human melanoma defined by a precipitating antibody in human serum. Int.

J. Cancer 32:717-721, 1983.

36. Giacomini P., Aguzzi A., Fisher P.B. and Ferrone S. Modulation by DNA recombinant immune interferons of the synthesis, expression and shedding of tumour associated antigens by human melanoma cells. Submitted, 1984.

37. Giacomini P., Aguzzi A. and Ferrone, S. Differential effect of recombinat immune interferon on the two subunits of Class I HLA antigens and induction of a 14K polypeptide. In preparation.

38. Giacomini P., Aguzzi A. and Ferrone S. Class II HLA antigens and melanoma: Differential susceptibility of gene products of the HLA-D region to modulation by recombinant immune interferon. Submitted, 1984.

39. Natali P.G., Cavaliere R., Matsui M., Buraggi G., Callegaro L. and Ferrone S. Human melanoma associated antigens identified with monoclonal antibodies: characterization and potential clinical application. Submitted, 1984.

40. Imai K., Natali P.G., Kay N.E., Wilson B.S. and Ferrone S. Tissue distribution and molecular profile of a differentiation antigen detected by a monoclonal antibody (345.134S) produced against human melanoma cells. Cancer Immunol. & Immunother. 12:159-166, 1982.

41. Imai K., Wilson B.S., Bigotti A., Natali P.G. and Ferrone S.A. 94,000 Dalton glycoprotein expressed by human melanoma and carcinoma cells. J. Natl. Cancer. Inst. 68:761-769, 1982.

42. Liao S.K., Clarke B.J., Khosravi M., Kwong P.C., Brickenden A. and Dent P.B. Human melanoma-specific oncofetal antigen defined by a mouse monoclonal antibody. Int. J. Cancer 30:573-580, 1982.

43. Houghton A.N., Esinger M., Albino A.P., Cairncross J.G. and Old L.J. Surface antigens of melanocytes and melanomas:

Markers of melanocyte differentiation and melanoma subsets. J. Exp. Med. 156:1755, 1982.

44. Carrel S., Heumann P., Sekaly P., Zaech P., Buchegger F. and Girardet C. Characterization of a monoclonal antibody (A12) that defines a human acute lymphoblastic leukemia associated differentiation antigen. Hybridoma. In press. 1983.

45. Metzgar R.S. and Oleinick S.R. The study of normal and malignant cell antigens by mixed agglutination. Cancer Res. 28:1366–1371, 1968.

46. Zweig S.E. and Shevach E.M. Production and properties of monoclonal antibodies to guinea pig Ia antigens. Meth. in Enzymol. 92:73–74, 1983.

47. Laemmli, U.K. Cleavage of structural proteins during the assembly of the head of bacteriophage T4. Nature, 227:680–685, 1970.

48. Hunter W.M. and Greenwood F.C. Preparation of iodine–131 labelled human growth hormone of high specific activity. Nature 194:145–146, 1962.

Antimelanoma Monoclonal Antibodies in Immunoscintigraphy. Criteria for a Clinical Trial of the Italian National Research Council (C.N.R.)

Siccardi G.S.

Universita di Milano
Dipartimento di Biologia e Genetica
Via G.B. Viotti 5, 20133 Milano, Italy.

The Italian National Research Council has launched, a few years ago, a series of "Special Projects" with the aim to enhance the technological level of Italian industrial production through collaborative research and development programmes on projects of public utility in several fields, including the biomedical area. Such programmes involve the participation and direct collaboration of different Operative Units in Universities, Industry and other Institutions.

The Special Project "Biomedical Engineering", led by Prof. L. Donato, started its second five-year term in 1983. In its first five-year term, the Special Project had been instrumental in the introduction and development in Italy of a number of technologies and instrumentations, mainly related to artificial organs, nuclear magnetic resonance, bio-reactors, diagnostics etc.

In the present term, the Special Project "Biomedical Engineering" has recognized tumour immunoscintigraphy by means of monoclonal antibodies as a major objective and has launched collaborative programmes with a number of basic research and nuclear medicine units, in Italy and abroad, with the aim to assess the feasibility to produce and utilize bulk products of pharmaceutical quality derived from murine monoclonal antibodies. By radiopharmaceutical quality we mean consistent and reproducible reagents which can be routinely used in any nuclear medicine center, with a predictable bio-distribution and known reliability of tumour localization, using standard nuclear medicine procedures.

Melanoma, Colorectal carcinoma and Lung microcitoma Projects were started in 1982, 1983 and 1984, respectively, and are now at different stages of development. The Melanoma Project, the most advanced of the three programmes, was chosen as a pilot project for a number of reasons, including the tumour's rich vascularization, which allows an easy access for the antibodies from the blood stream, and the ease with which biopsies can be obtained from visible subcutaneous localizations, thus allowing immunocytochemical controls.

The industrial partner in the project, Sorin Biomedica, is the largest manufacturer of radiopharmaceuticals in Italy and the only Italian firm producing monoclonal antibodies on an industrial scale. A network of collaborating research units was thus constructed to support the industrial partner with the necessary expertise in basic research, clinical pathology, laboratory and nuclear medicine (Table 1).

The strategy adopted was to construct an "industrial processor" to transform a research reagent into a product for routine use, with all the characteristics appropriate to this kind of product in terms of reproducibility, safety and ease of utilization.

Such a strategy is illustrated by the sequential list of the steps which were dealt with, in sequence (Table 2).

TABLE 1 - OPERATIVE UNITS OF THE MELANOMA PROJECT.

Ferrone S.
Department of Microbiology and Immunlogy
New York Medical College
Valhalla, New York (U.S.A.)

Buraggi G.L.
Nuclear Medicine Department
National Tumours Institute
Milano, Italy

Mariani G.
Metabolism Department
Institute of Clinical Physiology of National Council
Pisa, Italy

Callegaro L.
Chemistry & Radiochemistry Research Department
Sorin Biomedica S.p.A.
Saluggia, Italy

Natali P.G.
National Tumour Institute
Regina Elena
Roma, Italy

TABLE 2 - MAIN STEPS OF THE MELANOMA PROJECT

1 - Choice of appropriate Mab's
2 - Radio-labelling of Mab and fragments
3 - Biodistribution studies (in patients bearing non-
   melanoma tumours)
4 - Radio-immuno-detection of tumour masses in melanoma
   patients
5 - Double-labelling experiments in vivo
6 - Immunohistochemistry studies on excised tumours
7 - Development of radiopharmaceuticals of industrial quality
8 - Development of an "instant-labelling" kit (Technemab-1)
9 - Evaluation of pilot tests (30 cases, stage III-IV patients)
10 - Multicenter Clinical Trial (10 Italian centers)
11 - Extension of the procedure to stage II patients without
   age limit
12 - Extension of Multicenter Clinical Trial to European
   Centers

The choice of the appropriate monoclonal antibody (Mab) is obviously a critical step. In the case of the Melanoma Project the Mab's were supplied by Ferrone, who had extensively characterized a set of reagents specific for a number of melanoma-associated-antigens, together with Natali and others (1,2). The same "high molecular weight" melanoma associated antigen could be identified by two monoclonals specific for two distinct epitopes. Such a marker is absent in normal tissues, with the exception of a few cells in the hair follicle, but it is detectable in the serum of normal individuals, as well as in melanoma patients, as documented by Giacomini et al. (3). The serum levels are very low and not significantly different in normal controls and tumour patients.

Localization studies of monoclonal antibody 225.28 S were carried out by Those, Ferrone et al. (4) in nude mice grafted with human melanoma. The choice of the Mab and/or $F(ab')_2$ fragments to be used in human melanoma patients was eventually decided by immunoreactivity and stability studies of radiolabelled material as well as by biodistribution studies in patients with tumours other than melanoma (5).

The radio-labelling of these monoclonal antibodies and of their $F(ab')_2$ fragments was carried out by Callegaro et al. (6,7). It is worth stressing that each Mab is an homogeneous reagent of its own, and that its chemical handling and its labelling properties might thus present unpredictable characteristics.

The biodistribution of labelled reagents represents the only real operative criterium which can be studied prior to the evaluation of tumour localization in humans. Aspecific homing of labelled monoclonal antibodies or fragments in various organs has been documented by many authors; in most cases it is very difficult to established how " aspecific" such homing is, since the nominal antigen or cross-reacting antigens or immune complexes might be localized in the target organs. The fraction of aspecific homing which disappears using fragments instead of intact immunoglobulins is assumed to be due to Fc-receptor activity. Pilot studies in animal systems by Spira et al. (8) demonstrate that mutant monoclonal immunoglobulins, deleted in various Fc domains, show a different distribution to the original reagent. Since such mutants can be screened among the mutagenized progeny of any hybridoma cell line, these findings offer possible interesting developments to enhance the operative value of reagents with

207

H

interesting antibody specificities, but poor biodistribution properties. A particular case is represented by IgM reagents, which seem to circulate very well but are ineffective in tumour localization. In this case the problem might be difficulty in leaving the blood stream to reach tissue targets.

Again, the in-vitro attainment of "switch variants" of IgG isotype with the same paratopic specificity as the original IgM might allow the clinical use of reagents of interesting specificity but of unsuitable isotype. A new Operative Unit of our Project will start work later this year, in this direction, i.e. the development of suitable mutant immunoglobulins.

Studies of the biodistribution of labelled reagents in patients with tumours other than melanoma were carried out by Mariani et al. (5,9) and demonstrated that, in the case of the Mab 225.28 S, F(ab')$_2$ fragments had a much better "in-vivo behaviour" than the intact immunoglobulins.

The pilot study to evaluate the localization of melanoma lesions was conducted by Buraggi et al. (10,11). Different labels were tested in sequence (^{131}I, ^{99m}Tc, ^{111}In) and the results compared according to various parameters (11). Since a good proportion of the known lesions was actually imaged, in spite of variable but consistent background localizations, a number of controls were set up to evaluate the sensitivity, the specificity and the reliability of the diagnostic procedure. The controls included a comparison between the distribution of the specific reagent and that of aspecific reagents (irrelevant monoclonal antibodies of the same isotype but labelled with another isotope, ^{99m}Tc-Pertechnetate, ^{99m}Tc-labelled albumin) (11,12). The controls also included, whenever possible, the immunohistochemical analysis of the excised tumour tissues with a panel of different monoclonal antibodies (1). Although the problem of background localization is far from being solved and although the correlation between radioactivity accumulation and melanotic lesions may vary considerably in various organs and anatomical regions, the overall results are very encouraging. Above 70 % of known lesions have been visualized, while many previously unknown lesions which were visualized by this technique were subsequently confirmed by other methods and/or by surgery.

The development of an "instant labelling" kit Technemab-1 (7) enabled us to extend the test to a number of Nuclear Medicine Centers in Italy, and to start a Multicenter Clinical Trial (Table 3), where all participants could use exactly the same reagents without any logistical problem and could follow a common Immunoscintigraphy Protocol, the same accepted by the Ethical Committee of the Instituto Nazionale Tumori of Milan for the pilot study of Buraggi et al (Table 4). Local difficulties to obtain the necessary clearance for the human clinical trials have in some cases delayed the actual start of the programme, but now all the listed groups are active and have studied a significant number of cases. Up to now, more than 150 cases have been studied by using different isotopes, but mainly ^{99m}Tc.

Only at the end of the year will we be able to summarize the results obtained, but it is quite clear that in all centers which have performed a certain number of cases (20 or above), the results are similar to those obtained in the pilot study (12).

The Ethical Committee of the Istituto Nazionale Tumori of Milan, having realized the absence of any adverse reactions following the diagnostic procedure, has recently given its clearance to extend the procedure to less "terminal" patients, thus allowing a considerable broadening of the patient population to which the procedure can be applied. At the same time other centers in Europe have been included in the Multicenter Trial and have already started to work.

TABLE 3 -
ITALIAN MULTICENTER CLINICAL TRIAL

Abbati A.
Nuclear Medicine Division
O¬pedale Maggiore
Bologna

Riva P.
Nuclear Medicine Division
Ospedale Bufalini
Cesena

Bestagno M.
Nucelar Medicine Division
Spedali Civili
Brescia

Salvatore M.
Tumour Institute
Fondazione Pascale
Napoli

Galli G.
Nuclear Medicine Institute of
Catholic University
Roma

Sanguineti M.
Nuclear Medicine Division
Ospedale Galliera
Genova

Masi R.
Nuclear Medicine Division
Ospedale Careggi
Firenze

Turco G.L.
Nuclear Medicine Institute of
Turin University
Torino

TABLE 4 -

SCHEME OF THE IMMUNOSCINTIGRAPHY CLINICAL PROTOCOL

1. Criteria for patient selection.

Reference is made to the clinical classification by Stehling (1963), in use of the Anderson Hospital.

a) (At the beginning of the study). Stage IV patients, without age limits. Stage IIIB, or IIIAB, of age above 65, with regional metastases, including cutaneous and subcutaneous ("in transit") lesions beyond 3cm from the primitive lesions.

b) (Since recently). Patients suffering from malignant melanoma with local, regional or distant recurrences, hospitalized for adequate staging and therapy. Also Stage II are considered, without age limits. The patients should not show severe changes in laboratory findings.

2. History of allergy.

Patients suffering from atopic or allergy diseases, including contact dermatitis and hypersensitivity to radiopaque agents, were excluded from the study.

3. Informed Consent

4. Patient preparation and safety requirements.

a) Treatment with Lugol's solution 2% (20 drops orally, twice daily for 3 days), for patients to be treated with Iodine-labelled radiopharmaceuticals. Treatment with potassium perchlorate (400 mg) 30-60 min prior to injection for patients to be treated with Technetium-labelled radiopharmaceuticals.

b) Immediate-type hypersensitivity intradermic test (0.1 ml

mouse IgG, 35 ug/ml in isotonic saline, and 0.1 ml isotonic saline in the controlateral arm) 30 min prior to injection.

c) Ready availability of an intensive care specialist must be guaranteed at the moment of injection.

5. Laboratory analyses.

a) Complete blood count, platelets count and ESR.

b) Liver and renal function tests.

c) Plasma electrolytes levels.

d) Electrophoresis and immunodiffusion of serum proteins.

e) Blood glucose and cholinesterase.

f) Chest X-ray and ECG.

All to be performed in the week preceeding the injection and repeated one week after.

6. Immunocytochemistry. (whenever possible)

Immunoperoxidase staining on the excised tumour tissues, performed with the same Mab used for immunoscintigraphy and with two other anti-melanoma Mab's, specific for different epitopes.

REFERENCES

1) Natali P.G., Bigotti A., Cavaliere R., Nicotra M.R. and Ferrone S. Phenotype of lesions of melanocyte origin with monoclonal antibodies to melanoma associated antigens and to HLA antigens.

J. Natl. Cancer Inst. 73: 13-24, 1984.

2) Natali P.G., Cavaliere R., Bigotti A., Imai K., Nicotra M.R., Russo C., Ng A.K., Giacomini P. and Ferrone S. Antigenic heterogeneity of surgically removed primary and autologous

metastatic human melanoma.

J. Immunol., 130: 1462–1466, 1983.

3) Giacomini P., Veglia F., Còrdiali Fei P., Rehele T., Natali P.G. and Ferrone S. Level of membrane bound high molecular weight melanoma-associated antigen in patients with melanoma and of a cytoplasmic melanoma associated antigen in surgically removed tissues and in sera from patients with melanoma.

Cancer Res., 44: 1281–1287, 1984.

4) Glose T., Ferrone S., Imai K., Nowell S.T., Luner S.J., Martin R.H. and Blair A.H. Imaging of human melanoma xenografts in nude mice with a radiolabelled monoclonal antibody.

J. Natl. Cancer Inst. 69: 823–826, 1982.

5) Mariani G., Callegaro L., Mazzucca M., Macchia D., Mencaci S., Buraggi G.L., Ferrone S., Rosa U. and Bianchi R.

An in vivo study on the issue distribution of anti-human melnoma monoclonal antibodies.

J. Nucl. Med. All. Sci. 27, 148–150, 1983.

6) Callegaro L., Ferrone S., Plassio G., Dovis M., Mariani C., Buraggi G.L., Boniolo A. and Rosa U. Biochemical characterization of monoclonal antibodies and $F(ab')_2$ fragments against human melnoma associated antigen labelled with different radioactive isotopes.

J. Nucl. Med. All. Sci. 27, 82–85, 1983.

7) Callegaro L., Deleide G., Dovis M., Cecconato E., Plassio G. and Rosa U. Purification and labelling of $F(ab')_2$ fragments and their conversion to radiopharmaceuticals.

Proceedings of Saariselka Symposium 10–11 August 1983.

8) Spira G., Bargellesi A., and Scharff M.D. Selection of class-switch mutants by Sib-selection and ELISA.

J. Immunol. Methods, 1984, in press.

9) Mariani G. and Mazzucca M. Evaluation of the in-vivo distribution of radioiodinated monoclonal preparations as a screening procedure for potential tumour immunoscintigraphy agents.
Proceedings of Saariselka Symposium 10-11 August 1983.

10) Buraggi G.L., Callegaro L., Ferrone S., Turrin A., Cascinelli N., Attili A., Bombardieri E., Mariani G. and Deleide G. In-vivo immunodiagnosis with radiolabelled anti-melanoma antibodies and $F(ab')_2$ fragments.
Nuclear Medizin : Proceeding of the 21 Int. Ann. Meet. S.N.M.E., Ulm 13-16 Sept. 1983, Ed. Schmidt H.A.E. and Adam W.E. Schattauer Verlag, Stuttgart, N.Y., 1984, 713-716.

11) Buraggi G.L., Turrin A., Cascinelli N., Attili A., Bombardieri E. and Gasparini M. Immunoscintigraphy with melanoma monoclonal antibody.
Proceeding of Saariselka Symposium 10-11 August 1983.

12) Paganelli G., Riva P., Fiorentini V., Tison V., Landi G. and Amadori D. Immunoscintigraphy with 99mTc-labelled $F(ab')_2$ fragments of an antimelanoma monoclonal antibody.
Proceedings of Saariselka Symposium 10-11 August 1983.

Immunoscintigraphy with Antimelanoma Monoclonal Antibodies

Buraggi G.L.*, Turrin A.*, Cascinelli N.**, Attili A.**, Terno G.***, Bombardierei E.*, Gasparini M.*, Seregni E.*

   * Nuclear Medicine Division
  ** Clinical Oncology Division E
 *** Anaesthesiology and Intensive Care Division
    Istituto Nazionale Tumori – Milano (Italy)

INTRODUCTION

Several researches involving the production, the characterization and the utilization in clinical oncology of monoclonal antibodies (MoAb) to tumour associated antigens expressed by different tumours, are in progress at the Istituto Nazionale Tumori of Milano (INT).

After the considerable results obtain by Goldenberg et al (1), Mach et al (2), immunoscintigraphy, as a new approach to tumour imaging, was identified by our group as a priority research field. Experiments to study radioimmuno-localization in nude mice were performed with different monoclonal antibodies labelled with ^{131}I (3).

The first experiments with immunoscintigraphy in man performed by us were carried out in patients bearing malignant melanomas (4-7) with a monoclonal antibody to a human high molecular weight-melanoma associated antigen (HMW-MAA), previously studied by Ferrone, Natali et al (8, 9, 10, 11, 12 – 17, 18). The HMW-MAA is expressed by at least 90% of melanoma lesions (18), is undetectable in normal tissue except for hair follicles (10, 12, 16), is present only in minute amounts in serum (19) and is less heterogeneous in its expression than other types of melanoma-associated antigens (13).

Among the different monoclonal antibodies obtained by these Authors the MoAb 225-28S showed the most favourable characteristics for immunoscintigraphy.

It was also shown that ^{125}I-MoAb 225-28S localises in human melanomas transplanted into nude mice (20).

The radiolabelling procedures and the preparation of the whole MoAb 225-28S and its F(ab')2 fragments for injection in man were studied by Callegaro et al (21). Mariani et al (22, 23) studied the metabolic behaviour in patients bearing malignant diseases other than melanoma.

A series of patients bearing malignant melanomas was studied at the INT using the immunoreagents labelled with different radioisotopes (5,6).

This paper reports the results obtained until now, within the frame of Special Project "Biomedical Engineering" of the Italian National Research Council.

A multicenter clinical trial programme, coordinated by CNR is now in progress with the collaboration of other Nuclear Medicine Institutions.

MATERIALS AND METHODS

Further details of the characteristics of the MoAb 225-28S and the radiolabelling procedures are reported by Ferrone and Callegaro elsewhere in this volume.

TABLE 1 - CHARACTERISTICS OF LABELLED ANTIBODIES UTILIZED

IMMUNOREAGENT	PATIENTS n°	INJECTED ANTIBODY (μg) X̄	RANGE	SPECIFIC ACTIVITY (mCi/mg) X̄	RANGE	INJECTED ACTIVITY (mCi) X̄	RANGE
^{131}I-MoAb-AM	2	21	14-28	52.1	50.7-53.6	0.92	0.70-1.42
	2	695	640-750	695.0	1.1		
^{131}I-F(ab')2-AM	4	22	18-30	41.7	31.0-57.2	1.01	0.93-1.04
^{123}I-F(ab')2-AM	4	217	170-290	14.8	12.0-17.4	3.18	2.40-4.00
^{99m}Tc-F(ab')2-AM	6	160	80-200	46.9	40.0-64.0	7.49	4.48-8.50
^{111}In-F(ab')2-AM	6	37	32-40	51.0	50.0-55.0	2.16	0.92-4.56
	10	288	106-420	11.6	3.9-18.6		
^{131}I-F(ab')2-AHB$_s$	6	20	15-60	29.5	9.0-56.0	0.60	0.50-0.80

TABLE 2 - DOSIMETRY
(D_T = rad/mCi)

ORGAN	^{131}I-MoAb	^{131}I-F(ab')$_2$	^{123}I-F(ab')$_2$	^{99m}Tc-F(ab')$_2$	^{111}In-F(ab')$_2$
WHOLE BODY	0.70	0.40	0.03	0.00003	0.37
BONE MARROW	0.77	0.32	0.14	0.002	0.27
KIDNEYS	7.79	1.66	0.03	0.097	0.49
SPLEEN	25.00	10.01	0.60	0.030	2.45
LIVER	2.02	1.44	0.86	0.010	1.15
OVARY	0.02	0.003	0.002	0.0009	0.002
TESTICLE	0.002	0.0003	0.00001	0.00004	0.003

Five different radioimmunoreagents were employed in this study, namely ^{131}I-MoAb, ^{131}I-F(ab')2, ^{123}I-F(Ab')2, ^{99m}Tc-F(ab')2 and ^{111}In-F(ab')2. Table 1 summarizes the mean value and the range of the principal parameters of the injected compounds in each group of patients. The last compound reported in the table was prepared by labelling the F(ab')2 fragments of an irrelevant antibody of the same isotype (HBsAg-MoAb 4C1) with ^{131}I and it was utilized to check the uptake specificity of the other compounds in neoplastic tissue.

Different imaging techniques (24) such as analogue and computerized scintigraphy, subtraction techniques, double antibody techniques and single photon emission tomography (SPECT) were employed. Behavioural studies of the different compounds in the whole body, in different organs and in tumours were performed with serial examinations by computerized scintigraphy (regional and whole body) using the ROI technique. Serial blood samples were drawn to study the behaviour of the compounds in the blood pool.

When surgical specimens of the tumours were available, in vitro radioactive measurements and immunostaining were performed. A protocol with suggestions and guidelines for the study was elaborated with the collaboration of different specialists and approved by the Research Committee of the INT. It was later adopted by CNR for the Multicenter Clinical Trials programme. Very strict criteria were established at the beginning of the study for patients' admission. Only patients with advanced malignant melanomas (stage IIIB and IIIAB aged more than 65 years and stage IV) were admitted.

Only after verifying the absence of adverse reaction was the study extended to all stages. Clinical analyses for the evaluation of hepatic, pancreatic, hematopoietic and renal functions were performed in all patients before the injection and repeated 4 times in the following 2 weeks.

Informed consent, no previous allergic diseases, no reaction to the skin test were other most important criteria for admission.

The injection of the immunoreagents was always performed in the presence of an intensive care specialist.

Whenever ^{131}I or ^{123}I tracers were used, thyroid uptake was blocked by potassium iodide, 120 mg/day for 10 days, starting 3 days before the injection.

When ^{99m}Tc tracer was used, thyroid blocking was obtained by administered 400 mg of potassium perclorate to the patients before the injection.

RESULTS

From May 1982 to June 1984, 34 patients bearing malignant melanomas were examined.

Neither immediate adverse reactions or evident modifications of the functional analyses performed before and after the injection of the immunoreagents were observed. The amount of the injected antibody was usually low with a relatively high specific activity (Table 1). In some cases, higher amounts of the antibody with low specific activity were used but no consistent difference was observed in tumour fixation, nor in the body distribution of the two groups of reagents. The amount of radioactivity to be injected was chosen according to the dosimetry calculated for each radionuclide. In the case of the reagent used, a consistent difference in body distribution was observed between the whole antibody and the F(ab')2 fragment. Fig. 1 shows the disappearance curves obtained in 2 patients injected with the whole immunoglobulin (panel a) or the fragments (panel b). In both cases the antibodies were labelled with ^{131}I and the curves were corrected for the decay.

DISAPPEARANCE CURVES OF ^{131}I-MoAb 225.285

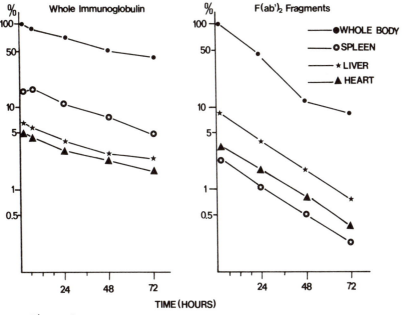

Figure 1

The whole antibody disappears from the whole body, blood pool, spleen and liver more slowly than the F(ab')2 fragments. In the former case this results, on the one hand, in a very high background and, on the other, in a higher irradiation of the patient. For these reasons any further study was performed with F(ab')2 fragments.

To improve technical scintigraphic conditions and to reduce the irradiation of the patients, ^{123}I, ^{99m}Tc and ^{111}In were used.

Fig. 2 reports the mean values of the blood clearance of the five reagents obtained by the study of 4 patients in each group.

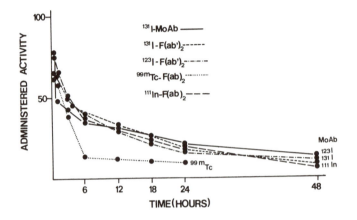

BLOOD CLEARANCE OF ANTI-MELANOMA MONOCLONAL
ANTIBODIES: CUMULATIVE RESULTS.

Figure 2

The most considerable difference is shown by the technetium compound which decreases very rapidly in the first few hours after injection. There is probably a release of technetium (free or bound to small fragments) from the compound. This fact is confirmed by an early visualization of urinary tract and also by the behaviour of the disappearance curve from the whole body and from various organs, which are reported in Fig. 3 and which were obtained by the study of 3-5 patients of each group.

When compared to the other tracers, the indium compound

222

shows an increased activity in the liver and also, to a lesser extent, in the bone marrow. Even in this case a release of the radionuclide is possible.

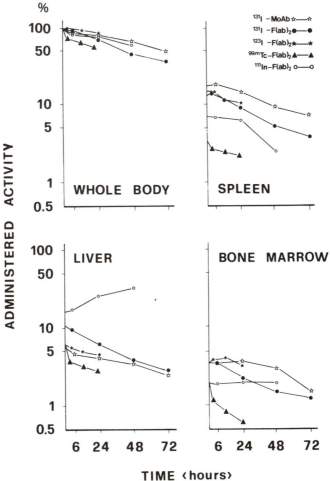

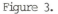

Figure 3.

Main disappearance curves from whole body and various organs of antimelanoma MoAb and $F(ab')_2$ fragments labelled with different radioisotopes.

As a general remark, the persistence of radioactivity in the abdominal organs, namely liver and spleen, represents, from a scintigraphic point of view, the most noticeable disadvantage. The results of dosimetric evaluations for the five compounds are reported on Table 2. Mean clearance curves from whole body and from single organs were utilized for calculation, according to the suggestion of Medical International Radiation Dose Committee (25).

There is a big difference between the compounds labelled with ^{131}I and the other compounds. Among these ^{99m}Tc offers the most favourable conditions, followed by ^{123}I and ^{111}In. A not negligeable dose to spleen and liver is due to the latter. As to tumour accumulation, we did not observe any significant difference between the five compounds used. In the positive cases tumour uptake is evident from the very first minutes after injection, as is shown in Fig. 4.

This rapid uptake is probably connected with a high degree of vascularisation of neoplastic tissue. The maximum value of tumour/background ratio is reached at different times after injection and differs not only from patient to patient but, sometimes, even among the various lesions in the same patient (Fig.5).

The evaluation of the variations versus the time of the mean value of tumour/background ratio and the range of variation in the whole series of patients examined lead to some practical suggestions concerning the use of the immunoreagent.

As shown in Fig 6, the best conditions to carry out immunoscintigraphy study are normally reached from 6 to 24 hours after injection.

As reported, the vascularization of the tumours must play an important role in the uptake of the antibody by the neoplastic tissue. To check the specificity of antibody uptake by the tumours we carried out some experiments.

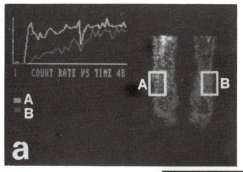

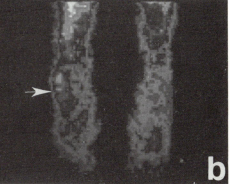

Figure 4.

Patient at stage IIIAB with a subcutaneous localization (4 cm) at the right ankle. Examination performed during 4 min after injection of 8 mCi (80 ug) of ^{99m}Tc-F(ab')$_2$. Panel a shows the ROIs curves in the tumour area (A) and in a normal symmetrical area. Panel b shows the picture resulting from the sum of the 48 frames used to obtain the ROIs curves. It can be seen that from the very first minutes the accumulation rate in the tumour is higher than in the symmetrical area. In this early phase radioactivity is present also in vascular and interstitial spaces of the legs, from where it disappears after 1–2 hours.

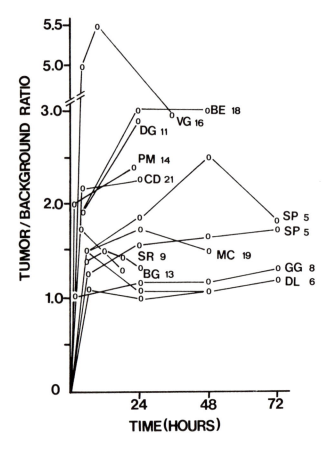

Figure 5.

Variation with time of tumour/background ratio in a group of patients.

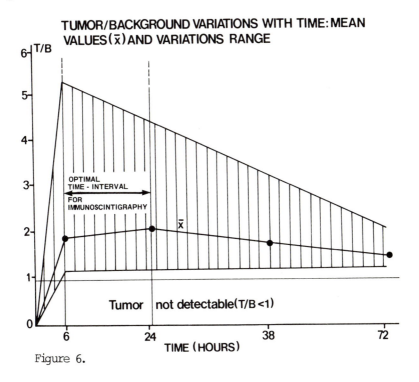

TUMOR/BACKGROUND VARIATIONS WITH TIME:MEAN
VALUES($\bar{x}$)AND VARIATIONS RANGE

Figure 6.

Injecting in the same patient the immunoreagent labelled with ^{99m}Tc and, after 3 days, ^{99m}Tc pertechnetate, a very different distribution of radioactivity was observed in the tumour area: 1 hour after the injection of the antibody, the tumour was imaged as an isolated area, whereas after the same interval of time, pertechnetate was distributed in the whole region.

After simultaneous injection of the anti-melanoma f(ab')2, labelled with ^{99m}Tc or ^{111}In, and of an irrelevant F(ab')2 (Table

227

1), tumour/background (T/B) ratios were evaluated in 4 patients by "in vivo" measurements and, in 1 case, also by measurements of surgical specimens.

The values of T/B ratios of the specific F(ab')2 were always higher (1.3 - 1.9 times) than those of the irrelevant F(ab')2. These results were confirmed by the immunoscintigraphy performed in the two different measurement conditions.

In our study several scintigraphic techniques were utilized to obtain the best conditions in tumour imaging, but the variety of neoplastic localization in advanced melanoma do not allow general suggestions.

Conventional techniques are usually sufficient for a good demonstration of peripheral localization, as it can be seen in Fig. 7, which refers to 2 patients with neoplastic localizations respectively to the groin (panel a) and foot (panel b). Moreover they are aften sufficient in more complex situations, such as in the case reported in Fig. 8. This patient had a malignant pleural effusion with complete radiological opacity: the map shows a diffuse irregular accumulation of the radioactivity in the right hemithorax.

Sometimes a subtraction technique may be useful to better define the extent of a lesion. To avoid a misinterpretation of possible artefacts, we utilize this technique only if tumour is seen on conventional maps.

Single photon emission tomography (SPECT) can be very useful to allow the isolated representation of a tumour and improved the scintigraphic resolution (Fig. 9).

The interpretation of the results obtained by immunoscintigraphy requires, as reported, the evaluation of the specificity of the immunoreagent uptake by the tumour. Moreover it is important to verify whether and at which level the tumour explored expresses the H M W–M A A.

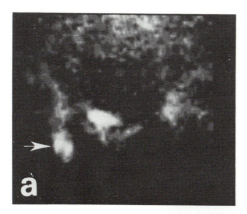

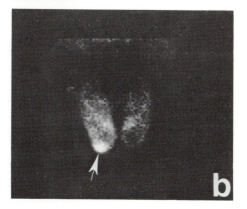

Figure 7.

Panel a: patient at stage III with a metastatic localization (4 cm) to the right groin. Immunoscintigraphy performed 4 hours after injection of 2.4 mCi (200 ug) of ^{123}I-F(ab')$_2$.

Panel b: patient at stage I with a primary melanoma (3 cm) to the right heel. Immunoscintigraphy performed 23 h after injection of 2 mCi (100 ug) of ^{111}In–F(ab')$_2$.

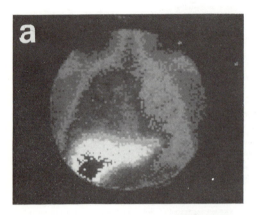

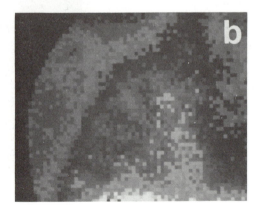

Figure 8.

Patient at stage IV with right malignant pleural effusion examined 48 hours after injection of 2.4 mCi (70 ug) of ^{111}In: standard projection (panel a) and magnification (panel b).

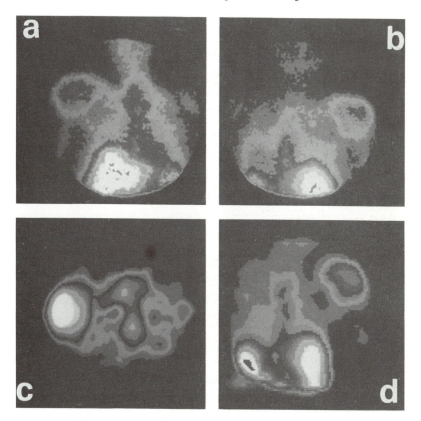

Figure 9.

Patient at stage IV with metastatic deposit to the right shoulder involving regional bones and soft tissues. Scintigraphic examinations performed 4 hours after injection of 3.3 mCi (320 ug) and ^{111}In-F(ab')2. Conventional projection (a, b) allow the demonstration of the lesion which is better studied with the other thoracic regions with emission tomography (SPECT): c=transversal and d=coronal projections.

A very useful technique to check this behaviour is the avidinbiotin immunoperoxidase staining of surgical specimens removed from the patients examined.

This method was currently applied by us whenever a patient was operated (Fig. 10).

Fig. 11 shows a correlation between scintigraphy, staining and lesion size in 15 lesions which could be examined. From this comparison it can be concluded that no false positive results were evident, i.e. no positive scintigraphies with negative staining. Two cases were negative with both methods, i.e. true negative. All the other lesions were positive to staining, but about half were negative to scintigraphic examination. Even if some of the latter had a small size, the others had larger dimensions, certainly sufficient for scintigraphic demonstration.

The cumulative results of this study are reported in Fig. 12. Positive results were obtained in 68,70% of all lesions examined. No false positive results were observed. There is a correlation between lesion size and positivity. Even if some lesions with a diameter of 1 cm or less could be visualized, a remarkable increase of positivity (up to 80%) was reached if lesions of 2 cm or more were considered. A correlation is also evident with the site, superficial or deep, of a lesion. Fig. 13 shows the increased incidence of positive results obtained considering all lesions of different size compared with the superficial ones. It can be observed that both lines increase rapidly to reach 100% for lesions of 3 cm, which can therefore be assumed as the threshold of a

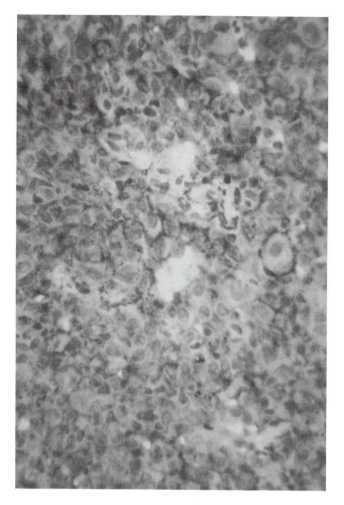

Figure 10.

Immunoperoxidase staining in a metastatic nodule of a malignant melanoma. Brown colour corresponds to antibodies fixed to cellular surfaces. This localization was positive at immunoscintigraphy.

Figure 11.

CORRELATION BETWEEN IMMUNOSCINTIGRAPHY (SC),
IMMUNOSTAINING (ST) AND LESION SIZE IN 15
LESIONS EXAMINED.

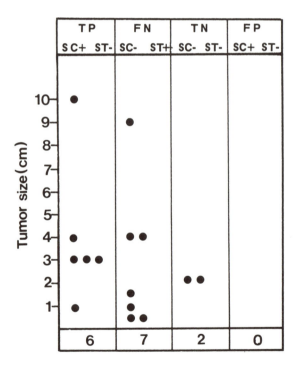

complete positive detection with respect to lesion size. Nevertheless among lesions of 3 and 8 centimeters there is a lack of positivity which is only partially due to the depth of the lesion. If we consider that a good reactivity of the antibody with the neoplastic tissues was found by immunostaining in about 90% of the cases examined, it is probable that the lack of visulization of the tumour is mostly due to local unfavourable anatomical conditions, such as bad vascularization, which does not allow the antibody to reach the tumour itself.

Figure 12. **CORRELATION BETWEEN SCINTIGRAPHIC REPRESENTATION AND SIZE OF 64 TUMOR LOCALIZATIONS IN 34 PATIENTS EXAMINED**

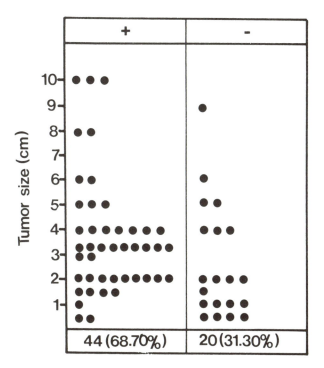

235

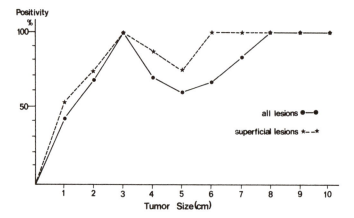

CORRELATION BETWEEN SCINTIGRAPHIC POSITIVITY AND SIZE IN ALL (64)
LOCALIZATIONS AND IN SUPERFICIAL (47) LESIONS

Figure 13.

DISCUSSION

This study has shown that the MoAb 225-28S labelled with different radioisotopes can be considered a radiopharmaceutical suitable for immunoscintigraphy of malignant melanomas.

The distribution of F(ab')2 fragments in the human body is more favourable than that of the whole immunoglobulin. Positive results were obtained in about the 70% of the neoplastic localizations examined.

This figure increased to 80%, if only lesions with a diameter of 2 cm or more were considered. A correlation with the depth of the lesions was also found. It was estimated that, from a geometrical point of view, a complete positivity can be reached with a lesion size of 3 cm irrespective of its location. Other factors affect the outcome of immunoscintigraphy, such as the level of expression of HMW-MAA and the regional anatomical conditions probably involving the vascularization of tumourous tissue.

Indeed, when comparative studies by immunoscintigraphy and immunohistochemical analysis were performed, all tumours imaged showed positive staining. In 2 localizations, where the HMW-MAA was not expressed, immunoscintigraphy was negative.

On the other hand, a significant number of lesions, which expressed the HMW-MAA, were not imaged as if the injected MoABwas unable to reach them.

The specificity of tumour uptake of the MoAb 25-28S was confirmed by the behaviour of a vascular-interstitial tracer like ^{99m}Tc-pertechnetate, on the one hand, and of an irrelevant ^{131}I-F(ab')2 of the same isotype, on the other hand.

A very different distribution in tumour and in the surrounding area was found in both cases.

The accumulation of the specific MoAb, in case of positivity, starts from the first minutes after injection. The study of tumour/background ratio in relation to time allowed to establish that the best conditions to perform immunoscintigraphy are normally reached from 6 to 24 hours after injection.

As to the choice of the radioisotope to obtain the best conditions for a routine examination, several factors must be considered.

From a dosimetric point of view, the technetium compound is the most favourable, followed by ^{123}I. Both these radioisotopes

237

have an optimal gamma emission energy for imaging instrumentation. The preparation of the immunoreagent in a lyophilised form, studied by Callegaro and his group, allows the labelling with ^{99m}Tc in a very simple way. The only limitation of this reagent is associated to a release of about 10% technetium, free or bound to smaller fragments of the protein molecule. This phenomenon is observed immediately after injection, it does not seem to interfere with the tumour imaging but leads to an increased background resulting from the visualization of the urinary tract. The indium compound gives the possibility of prolonging the study for a longer interval of time; however it too shows a certain release, demonstrated by a higher accumulation in liver and bone marrow. The dosimetry is less favourable and therefore a lower amount of radioactivity can be injected.

The accumulation of the technetium compound in various organs, namely liver, spleen, bone marrow and kidney is at present the most important problem to be solved. Background decreases using the F(ab')2 fragments instead of the whole immunoglobulin, but further improvements would be desirable for the study of abdominal organs.

During this study no adverse reactions were observed nor late alterations of the different functional examinations performed after the administration of the MoAb.

Also other groups who are using different monoclonal antibodies to perform immunoscintigraphy in melanoma (26,27), in ovarian, breast and gastrointestinal tumours (28) or in colorectal carcinoma (29, 30, 31, 32, 33, 34, 35) made similar observations and this represents an important factor for the future of this technique.

REFERENCES

1. Goldenberg D.M., De Land F., Kim E., Bennet S., Primus F.J., Van Nagell J.R.,Estes N., De Simone P. and Rayburn P. Use of radiolabelled antibodies of CEA for the detection and localization of diverse cancers by external photoscanning.

N. Engl. J. Med. 298: 1384-1388, 1978.

2. Mach J.P., Forni M., Ritschard J., Buchegger F., Carrel S., Widgren S., Donath A. and Alberto P. Use and limitations of radiolabelled anti-CEA antibodies and their fragments for photoscanning detection of human colorectal carcinomas.

Oncodev. Biol. Med. 1, 49-69, 1980.

3. Menard S., Miotti S., Tagliablue E., Parmi L., Buraggi G.L. and Colnaghi M.I., Tumour radioimmunolocalization in a murine system using monoclonal antibodies.

Tumori, 69: 185:190, 1983.

4. Buraggi G.L., Callegaro L., Ferrone S., Turrin A., Cascinelli N., Attili A., Bombardieri E., Mariani G., Deleide G. In vivo immunodiagnosis with radiolabelled anti-melanoma antibodies and F(ab')2 fragments. Nuclear medizin: Proceedings of the 21 Int. Ann. Meet. S.N.M.E. Ulm 13-16 Sept. 1983, Ed Schattauer Verlag Stuttgart, N.Y., 1984, 713-716.

5. Buraggi G.L., Callegaro L., Mariani G., Turrin A., Cascinelli N., Attili A., Bombardieri E., Terno G., Plassio G., Dovis M., Mazzucca N., Natali P.G., Scassellati D., Rosa U. and Ferrone S. Imaging with ^{131}I-labelled monoclonal antibodies to a high molecular weight-melanoma associated antigen in patients with melanoma efficacy of whole Ig and its Fab_2 fragments. Submitted for publication 1984.

6. Buraggi G., Callegaro L., Turrin A., Cascinelli N., Attili A., Emanuelli H., Gasparini M., Deleide G., Plassio G., Dovis M.,

Mariani G., Natali P.G. and Ferrone S. Immunoscintigraphy with ^{123}I, ^{99m}Tc and ^{III}In-labelled Fab$_2$ fragments of monoclonal antibodies to a human high molecular weight melanoma associated antigen (HMW-MAA). Submitted for publication 1984.

7. Buraggi G.L., Turrin A., Ferrone S., Cascinelli N., Attili A., Ringhini R., Bombardieri E., Rodiari A., Scaiano D., Seregni E., Gasparini M., Villa M. Immunodiagnosis with radiolabelled anti-melnoma monoclonal antibodies and F(ab')2 fragments (Abstract)

Eur. J. Nucl. Med. 5, A. 18, 1983.

8. Ferrone S., Giacomini P., Natali P.G., Ruiter D., Buraggi G.L., Callegaro L., Rosa U. A human high molecular weight melanoma associated antigen (HMW-MAA) defined by monoclonal antibodies: A useful marker to raioimage tumour lesions in patients with melanoma. First Internat. Meet. on Boron Mutron Capture M.I.T. Boston 12-14 October 1983 pag. 174-183.

9. Imai K., Natali P.G., Kay N.E., Wilson B.S. and Ferrone S. Tissue distruption and molecular profile of a differentiationantigen detected by a monoclonal antibody (345.134S) produced against human melanoma cells.

Cancer Immunol., 12: 159-166, 1982.

10. Imai K., Pellegrino M.A., Wilson B.S. and Ferrone S. Higher cytolytic efficiency of an IgG2a than of an IgG1 monoclonal antibody reacting with the same (or spatially close) determinant on a human high molecular weight melanoma associated antigen.

Cell. Immunol. 72: 239-247, 1982.

11. Imai K., Wilson B.S., Bigotti A., Natali P.G. and Ferrone S. A 94,000 dalton glycoprotein expressed by human melanoma and carcinoma cells.

J. Natl. Cancer Inst., 68: 761-769, 1982.

12. Natali P.G., Bigotti A., Cavaliere R., Nicotra M.R. and Ferrone S. Phenotype of lesions of melanocyte origin with monoclonal antibodies to melanoma associated antigens and to HLA antigens.

J. Natl. Cancer Inst. 73: 13–24, 1984.

13. Natali P.G., Cavaliere R., Bigotti A., Imai K., Nicotra M.R., Russo C., Ng A.K., Giacomini P. and Ferrone S. Antigenic heterogeneity of surgically removed primary and autologus metastatic human melanoma.

J. Immunol. 130: 1462–1466, 1983.

14. Natali P.G., Cavaliere R., Matsui M., Buraggi G.L., Callegaro L., and Ferrone S., Human melanoma associated antigens identified with monoclonal antibodies: characterization and potential clinical application. In: Cutaneous Melanoma and Precursor Lesions, 1984 In press.

15. Natali P., Giacomini P., Buraggi G.L., Cavaliere R., Bigotti A., Callegaro L. and Ferrone S., Serological and binding characteristics of a monoclonal antibody (MoAb) to a human high molecular weight-melanoma associated antigen (HMW-MAA) for tumour imaging. Proceedings in the 1st Int. Symp. on "Recent advances in tumour immunology: from oncogenes to tumour antigens". In press.

16. Natali P.G., Imai K., Wilson B.S., Bigotti A., Cavaliere R., Pellegrino M.A. and Ferrone S. Structural properties and tissue distribution of the antigen recognized by the monoclonal antibody 653.40S to human melanoma cells.

J. Natl. Cancer Inst. 67: 591–601.

17. Natali P.G., Wilson B.S., Imai K., Bigotti A. and Ferrone S. Tissue distribution, molecular profile and shedding of a cytoplasmic antigen identified by the monoclonal antibody 465.12S to human

melanoma cells.

Cancer Res. 42: 583-589, 1982.

18. Wilson B.S., Imai K., Natali P.G. and Ferrone S. Distribution and molecular characterization of cell-surface and a cytoplasmic antigen detectable in human melanoma cells with monoclonal antibodies.

Int. J. Cancer 28: 293-300, 1981.

19. Giacomini P., Veglia F., Cordiali Fei P., Rehele T., Natali P.G. and Ferrone S. Level of membrane bound high molecular weight melanoma associated antigen (MAA) and of a cytoplasmic melanoma associated antigen in surgically removed tissues and in sera from patients with melanoma.

Cancer Res., 44: 1281-1287, 1984.

20. Those T., Ferrone S., Imai K., Nowell. S.T., Luner S.J., Marin R.H. and Blair A.H. Imaging of human melanoma xenografts in nude mice with a radiolabelled monoclonal antibody.

J. Natl. Cancer Inst. 69: 823-826, 1982.

21. Callegaro L., Ferrone S., Plassio G., Dovis M., Mariani C., Buraggi G.L., Boniolo A., Rosa U. Biochemical characterization of monoclonal antibodies and F(ab')2 fragments against human melanoma associated antigen labelled with different radioactive isotopes.

J. Nucl. Med. All. Sci., 27: 82-85, 1983.

22. Mariani G., Callegaro L., Mazzucca M., Macchia D., Mencaci S., Buraggi G.L., Ferrone S., Rosa U., Bianchi R. An in vivo study on the tissue distribution of anti-human melanoma monoclonal antibodies.

J. Nucl. Med. All. Sci. 27, 148-150, 1983.

23. Mariani G., Callegaro L., Mazzucca N., Cecconato E., Molea N., Dovis M., Fusani L., Deleide G., Buraggi G.L. and

Bianchi R. Tissue distribution of radiolabelled anti-CEA monoclonal antibodies in man. "Protides of the Biological Fluids" 32nd, 1984.

24. DeLand F.H., Kim E.E., Simmons G. and Goldenberg D.M. Imaging approach in radioimmunodetection.

Cancer Res. 40: 3046-3049, 1980.

25. Snyder W.S., Ford M.R. Warner G.G. and Watson S.B. "S" absorbed dose per unit cumulated activity for selected radionuclides and organs. In MIRD Pamphlet No. 11. Society of Nuclear Medicine, New York, p. 1-257, 1975.

26. Larson S.M., Brown J.P., Wright P.W., Carrasquillo J.A., Hellstrom I. and K.E. Imaging of melanoma with ^{131}I labelled monoclonal antibodies.

J. Nucl. Med., 24: 123-129, 1983.

27. Larson S.M., Carrasquillo J.A., Krohn K.A., Brown J.P., McGuffin R.W., Ferens J.M., Graham M.M., Hill L.D., Beaumier P.L., Hellstrom K.E. and Hellstrom I. Localization of ^{131}I-labelled p97-specific Fab.2* fragments in human melanoma as a basis for radiotherapy.

J. Clin. Invest., 72: 2101-2114, 1983.

28. Epenetos A., Britton K.E., Mather S., Shepherd J., Granowska M., Taylor-Papadimitrion J., Nimmon C., Durhin H., Hawkins L.R., Malpas J.S. and Bodmer W.F. Targeting of Iodine-123-labelled associated monoclonal antibodies to ovarian, breast and gastrointestinal tumours.

Lancet, ii: 999-1004, 1982.

29. Buchegger F., Haskell C.M., Schreyer M., Scazziga B.R., Randin S., Carrel S. and Mach J.P. Radiolabelled fragments of monoclonal antibodies against carcinoembryonic antigen for localization of human colon carcinoma grafted into nude mice.

J. Exp. Med., 158: 413-427, 1983.

30. Buraggi G.L., Callegaro L., Turrin A., Gennari L., Bombardieri E., Gasparini M., Mariani G., Doci R., Regalia E. and Seregni E. Immunoscintigraphy of colorectal carcinoma: remarks about an ongoing clinical trial. Proceedings of the 22 Int. Ann. Meet. S.N.M.E., Helsinki, 13-17 Aug. 1984 in Press.

31. Chatal J.F., Saccavini J. C., Gumoleau P., Douillard J.Y., Curtel C., Kremer M., Le Mevel B. and Koprowski H. Immunoscintigraphy of colon carcinoma.

J. Nucl. Med. 25: 307-214, 1984.

32. Farrands P.A., Perkins A.C., Pimm M.V., Hardy J.D., Embleton J.J., Baldwin R.W. and Hardcastle J.D. Radioimmunodetection of human colorectal cancers by an anti-tumours monoclonal antibody.

Lancet, ii: 387-400, 1982.

33. Mach J.P., Buchegger F., Forni M., Ritschard J., Berche C., Lumbroso J.D., Schreyer M., Girardet C., Accolla L.S. and Carrel S. Use of radiolabelled monoclonal anti CEA antibodies for the detection of human carcinomas by external photoscanning and tomoscintigraphy.

Immunol. Today, 2: 239-269, 1981.

34. Mach J.P., Chatal J.F., Lumbroso J.D., Buchegger F., Forni M., Ritchard J., Berche C., Douillard J.Y., Carrel S., Herlyn M., Steplewski Z. and Koprowski H. Tumour localization in patients by radiolabelled monoclonal antibodies against colon carcinoma.

Cancer Res. 43: 5593-5600, 1983.

35. Moldofski P.J., Powe J., Mulhern C.B., Hammond N.D., Sears H.F., Gatenby R.A., Steplewski Z. and Koprowski H. Imaging with radiolabelled F(ab')2 fragments of monoclonal antibody in patient with gastrointestinal carcinoma.

Radiology, 149: 549–55, 1983.

CONSIGLIO NAZIONALE DELLE RICERCHE - C. N. R.
NATIONAL RESEARCH COUNCIL - C. N. R.

Progetto Finalizzato Tecnologie Biomediche   Nov. 1984
Special Project on Biomedical Engineering

CLINICAL RESEARCH PROTOCOL

IMMUNOSCINTIGRAPHY FOR DETECTION OF
‚KNOWN AND/OR OCCULT METASTASES OF MALIGNANT MELANOMA
THROUGH RADIOLABELLED ANTI-MELANOMA MONOCLONAL ANTIBODIES

Investigators

G. L. Buraggi, A. Turrin, E. Bombardieri, M. Gasparini, R. Ringhini, E. Seregni -
Nuclear Medicine Dept, Istituto Nazionale per lo Studio e la Cura dei Tumori,
Milan

N. Cascinelli, A. Attili, F. Belli - Oncology Clinic "E", Istituto Nazionale per lo
Studio e la Cura dei Tumori, Milan

L. Callegaro, U. Rosa - Research Dept, SORIN Biomedica, Saluggia

H. Emanuelli, G. Terno - Anesthesiology Dept, Istituto Nazionale per lo Studio e
la Cura dei Tumori, Milan

M. Borroni - Health Physics Dept, Istituto Nazionale per lo Studio e la Cura dei
Tumori, Milan

ANTIMELANOMA M C A

1. **AIM OF THE STUDY**

The aim of the research is to confirm suspected metastases and/or to evidence occult localizations of malignant melanoma.

This clinical trial is essentially aimed at defining the test characteristics in terms of sensitivity and specificity through the use of a specific anti-melanoma monoclonal antibody or its $F(ab')_2$ fragments radiolabelled with different radioisotopes (131-I, 99m-Tc, 111-In).

Therefore, the data of clinical interest concern the correlation between scintigraphic results and actual presence or absence of disease, its localization and its extent.

The availability of histological samples tested by immunohistological methods may lead to more detailed information on the behaviour of the immunological reagent at foci level.

2. **DIAGNOSTIC STAGE**

2.1. **Patient selection**

Candidates for this study are patients affected by malignant melanoma with a local, regional or distant recurrence, admitted to hospital for suitable staging and subsequent therapy. These patients must not present severe alterations of results of exams in section 2.5.

2.2. **Allergological history**

Patients affected by allergic diseases, such as bronchial asthma, rhinitis, atopic eczema, alimentary or contact allergies or regressed allergies caused by drugs or iodinated contrast media, must be excluded from the study.

2.3. **Informed consent**

Each patient must be informed with clear and detailed information about the nature, aims and potential hazards of the clinical trial, and must consent to undergo administration of the radiopharmaceutical and subsequent performance of the test.

2.4. **Patient preparation**

When using radioiodine-labelled reagents, thyroid function should be inhibited through administration of 2% Lugol's solution (20 drops twice a day) starting 3 days before beginning antibody administration and continuing for one week after onset of therapy.

When 99m-Tc technetium is used, potassium perchlorate should be administered 30 - 60 min before i.v. injection (400 mg orally in single dose).

Patients should be skin tested for hypersensitivity to murine immunoglobulins prior to inoculation. Approximately 30 min prior to radiopharmaceutical injection, an intradermal skin test dose of 100 μl mouse $F(ab')_2$ (isotonic solution supplied on request together with the radiopharmaceutical) should be administered to fasting patients, simultaneously with a separate injection of an equivalent dose of isotonic saline in the contralateral arm. The skin test should be read at 20 min and if negative, the study should proceed and the radiopharmaceutical injected intravenously. At the time of injection, the availability of an emergency care specialist must be guaranteed for assistance and control of patients in case of adverse reactions.

2.5. Laboratory exams before radiopharmaceutical injection

Candidates for immunoscintigraphy with radiolabelled antibodies must undergo the following laboratory exams during the week before radiopharmaceutical administration.
a) complete blood count and platelet count
b) renal function tests
c) hepatic function tests
d) plasma electrolyte levels
e) electrophoresis and immunodiffusion of serum proteins
f) ESR
g) serum cholinesterase
h) blood glucose
i) ECG (plus cardiological examination if possible)
j) chest X-rays

2.6. Laboratory exams after radiopharmaceutical injection

The same laboratory exams performed before scintigraphy should be carried out also after scintigraphy.

3. OPERATIVE STAGE

3.1. Clinical status

The physician in charge, after analysing the results of laboratory exams (see enclosed patient's report form), should control the patient's vital signs prior to injection and again during administration.
Any sudden reaction must be recorded and cured. Any reactions and side effects occurring within 24 hours after injection must be recorded by the physician in charge.

3.2. Nuclear Medicine investigations

a) **Radiopharmaceutical:** anti-melanoma $F(ab')_2$ supplied by SORIN Biomedica S.p.A., Saluggia (Italy)
The monoclonal antibody fragments will be radiolabelled with different radioisotopes following standard protocols. The labelled fragments should be tested for immunoreactivity towards human melanoma cell lines.
Monoclonal antibody preparations should meet the following guidelines:
   - preparation under sterile conditions
   - final sterilization on 0.22 μm membrane filter
   - sterility test by standard culture techniques (U.S. Pharmacopeia)
   - pyrogen test by conventional methods
   - pharmaceutical grade final solution ready for i.v. injection.

b) **Administration technique:** i.v. injection

c) **In vivo investigations**
   - Each patient will undergo whole body scans to detect multiple localizations. Further imaging will be carried out on any area of particular interest by conventional techniques or SPECT.
   - Serial gamma-camera images will be obtained at different times, according to the radionuclide used as a tracer. The following times are suggested:

   131-I: 2, 6, 24, 48, 72, 96 hours

99m-Tc: 2, 6, 12, 24 hours

111-In: 2, 6, 24, 48, 72 hours

Occasionally, imaging may be performed at a later time.
Positive areas of uptake will be charted for surgical confirmation.

- Correlative imaging such as liver, spleen and bone scans (obtained with suitable radiolabelled agents) or blood pool imaging with 99m-Tc HSA will be performed to clarify questionable areas or improve detection by subtraction techniques.

- Serial blood samples will be obtained before injection at 5, 10, 20, 30, 60 min after injection, as well as at later times, whenever a whole body scan is performed (24, 48, 72 hours).

3.3. Histology tests (immunohistodiagnosis)

Whenever patients undergo therapeutic or palliative surgery, biopsy samples should be selected and the presence of lesions confirmed by:
a) gross radioactivity counts
b) immunoperoxidase staining for reactive antigen. When available, IgG's from different clones reactive for the same antigen (e.g. HMW melanoma-associated antigen) are tested on the same histological sample, to check the specificity of the immunoscintigraphy agent.

CHARACTERISTICS OF ADMINISTERED RADIOPHARMACEUTICAL

Name and Family Name ....

Number ....

Date ....

Lot no ....

Prepared dose, mCi ....

Residue, mCi ....

Radioactivity administered, mCi (°) ....

Specific activity, mCi/mg (°°) ....

Quantity administered, mg ....

Volume administered, ml ....

Radiopharmaceutical concentration administered, mCi/ml ....

(°)   evaluation through ionization chamber
(°°) value at the time of administration

IMMUNOSCINTIGRAPHY

EXAMS TO BE PERFORMED

BEFORE AND AFTER RADIOPHARMACEUTICAL ADMINISTRATION

Patient ....

Laboratory exams   Date ....

Blood count   **Hepatic function tests**

normal [   ]   pathological [   ]   normal [   ]   pathological [   ]

White cells ....   Neu ....   Total bilirubin ....
Red cells ....   Bas ....   Direct bilirubin ....
Hb ....   Eos ....   Indirect bilirubin ....
P ....   Mon ....   SGOT ....SGPT ....
Lymph ....   Ret ....   GT .... Prothrombin ....
                                          Alkaline phosphatase.............................
Renal function tests   LDH .... CPK ....
normal [   ]   pathological [   ]   Blood glucose ....
                                          Pre-operative CEA ....
Blood urea nitrogen ....
Blood creatinine ....   **Electrophoresis**
Blood uric acid ....   normal [   ]   pathological [   ]
Creat. clearance ....
Urinalysis ....   Proteins ....
           ....   Albumin ....
           ....   Globulins ....
           ....   A/G ratio ....

                                          Immunodiffusion
Plasma electrolyte levels   normal [   ]   .pathological [   ]
normal [   ]   pathological [   ]   IgA ....
                                          IgM ....
Na ....   Cl ....   IgG ....
K ....   Ca ....   ERS (1st hour) ....
Mg ....   Cu ....   Cholinesterase ....
P ....

250

ANTIMELANOMA M C A

PATIENT'S REPORT FORM

Hospital ....
....
Patient ....
Age, years .... Sex ☐ F ☐ M
Patient identification card, no ....
Date of exam ....
Primary tumour localization ....
Treated ☐ Non-treated ☐

Radionuclide ....
Antibody concentration administered, /ug ....
Radioactivity administered, mCi ....
Time interval between administration and scintigraphy ....
Scintigraphic technique employed
.   Scanner ☐
.   Gamma-camera ☐
.   Computer ☐
Special computing (subtraction, SPECT, etc.) - Specify ....
....

OBSERVATIONS

Adverse reactions ....
....
Problems ....
....
Diagnostic effectiveness ....
....
Other observations ....
....
....

Investigator's signature

....

One or more scintigraphic images should be enclosed.

SCHEME OF LOCALIZATIONS AND SCINTIGRAPHIC IMAGING

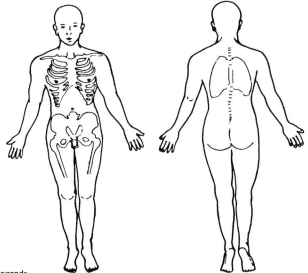

Legenda

0 = localization
1 = localization confirmed by scintigraphy
2 = occult localization evidenced by scintigraphy

CLINICAL STAGE ....

	Localizations	Dimensions	Scintigraphic result (+/-)
1	....	....	....
2	....	....	....
3	....	....	....
4	....	....	....
5	....	....	....

IN VITRO TESTS (immunoperoxidase staining)

1	....
2	....
3	....
4	....
5	....

ANTIMELANOMA M C A

BLOOD CLEARANCE CURVE

Name and Family Name ....
Number ....
Date ....

Sample collection	Time of administration, min	cpm
1		
2		
3		
4		
5		
6		
7		
8		
9		
10		

Melanoma Immunoscintigraphy with ^{99m} Tc-Labelled Monoclonal F(ab')$_2$: Sensitivity and Specificity Studies.

Riva P.[1], Paganelli G.[1]., Tison V.[2], Fiorentini G.[3], Landi G.[4], Amadori D.[5]

1. Servizio di Medicina Nucleare e Divisione Dermatologica[4] - Ospedale Generale Provinciale M. Bufalini, Cesena.
2. Instituto di Anatomia Patologica - Ospedale degli infermi, Faenza.
3. Divisione di Oncologia Medica - Ospedale S. Maria della Croci, Ravenna.
5. Centro Oncologica - Ospedale B. Morgagni, Forli

Thirty four cases of malignant melanoma (stages III and IV) have been studied using the instant labelling kit Technemab-1 developed by Sorin Biomedica (1) and tested by the pilot study of Buraggi (2,3) in the framework of the CNR Special Project "Biomedical Engineering"(4).

MATERIALS AND METHODS

Labelling was performed by addition of sterile and pyrogen-free ^{99m}Tc-pertechnetate to a lyophilized preparation (250 ug of F(ab')$_2$ fragments of the monoclonal antibody 225.28 S and by subsequent removal of free ^{99m}Tc by ion exchange column chromatography, according to the manufacturer's recommendations. The entire diagnostic procedure (patient selection and preparation, informed consent, laboratory tests etc.) was carried out following the Immunoscintigraphy Protocol of the CNR Multicenter Clinical Trial (4).

After the injection of the radiopharmaceutical (8-10 mCi), all patients were scanned at 4,8 and 24 hours post injection; imaging was also performed at other times with some of the patients. Blood samples were taken from all patients to evaluate (by paper chromatography) the percentage of free ^{99m}Tc, which varied progressively from < 3% (a few minutes after the injection) to approx. 20% (after 24 hours). Similar data was obtained in vitro from the radiopharmaceutical maintained in solution at ambient temperatures.

A large field of view gamma camera (Siemens) linked to a computer (Eurobit Sistema Idra) was employed for scanning and data processing.

SENSITIVITY

Out of 115 metastatic lesions documented by conventional methods (X rays, CT scans, ultrasonography etc.), 86 lesions (75%) were detected by immunoscintigraphy. Images obtained in different clinical situations and at different times after injection of the Tc-labelled anti-melanoma F(ab')$_2$ are reported in Fig. 1-3.

However, the sensitivity level obtained from our studies was not homogeneous. By analyzing the positive fraction in terms of size and organ localization (Table 1), it was found that only 30% of the lesions smaller than 2 cm were detected, while the degree of detection increased to 86%, when only lesions larger than 2 cm were considered. Moreover, brain, bone and lymph nodes localization were detected better than liver, lung and skin localizations. Three "negative" lesions were biopsied and tested by immunoperoxidase staining; two of them did not bind the antibody.

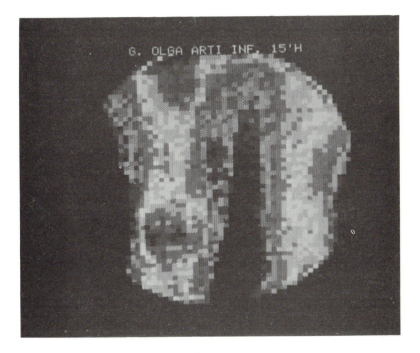

Figure 1 : Patient bearing multinodular localization on the right thigh and emolateral groin.

Processed image obtained 15 hrs. after i.v. injection.

257

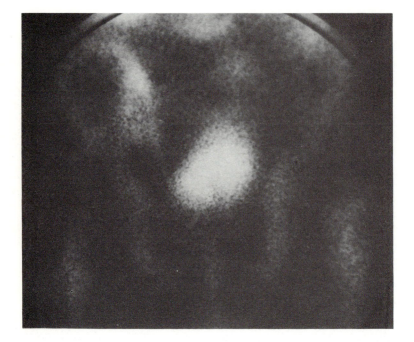

Figure 2 : Posterior scintigram of the pelvis performed 8 hrs. after i.v. injection. Bone metastases on the sacrumiliac joint and left iliac cresta are visualized.

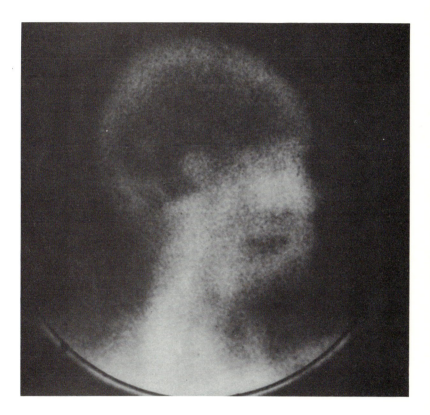

<u>Figure 3</u> : Right temporal and occipital metastatic sites of the brain.

Image obtained 4 hrs. after i.v. injection.

259

Table 1

Sensitivity of melanoma immunoscintigraphy (Tecnemab-1)

Organ	A No. of lesions	B No. (%) detected	C T/B ratio 8 hrs/24 hrs	D U.R.A.	E P/T
Liver	16	9 (56)	1.18/1.38	/	/
Lung	14	8 (57)	1.57/1.66	8	4/4
Bone	27	23 (85)	1.51/1.51	9	7/7
Brain	5	5 (100)	1.61/1.61	3	3/3
Superficial lymph nodes	25	20 (80)	2.25/2.16	3	3/3
Deep lymph nodes	7	6 (85)	1.91/2.10	9	2/3
Skin	12	8 (66)	2.00/2.50	5	4/4
Abdomen and pelvis	3	3 (100)	2.25/1.56	3	3/3
Other	6	4 (66)	1.80/1.96	/	/
Total	115	86 (75)	:::	40	25/26

A) Lesions documented by conventional methods

B) Lesions detected by immunoscintigraphy

C) Mean tumour/background ratio

D) Unexpected radioactivity accumulations

E) Lesions confirmed as metastases by other methods
(No positives/Not tested).

SPECIFICITY

Specificity controls were carried out in 7 patients who had shown positive scans with Tecnemab-1; four of them were subsequently injected with a comparable amount of ^{131}I-F(ab')$_2$ fragments of the monoclonal antibody 4B5, specific for HBsAg (supplied by Sorin Biomedica); three of them were subsequently injected with ^{99m}Tc-HSA (5 mg, 4 mCi). No positive scans were obtained in any of these cases. Fig 4 and 5 report a case, where right axillary lymph nodes were located with anti-melanoma monoclona F(ab')$_2$, whereas no radioactivity accumulation was seen with non specific F(ab')$_2$.

DISCUSSION AND CONCLUSIONS

As well as the 86 "positive" lesions an additional 40 radioactivity accumulations were recorded at sites where no metastatic lesions were known to exist. Figure 6 illustrates an unknown subcutaneous lesions 0.5 cm diameter on the left leg, confirmed by subsequent immunoperoxidase staining on bioptic tissue, obtained after surgery (Fig. 7).

Of such accumulations which could be investigated further (by follow-up, surgery, CT scans etc), 25 proved to be previously unknown metastatic lesions and only one was a "bona fide" false positive (an inflammatory lymph node). These findings, although hard to quantitate (since 14 cases out of 40 could not yet be investigated further) seem to be very promising for a use of immunoscintigraphy in prospective studies.

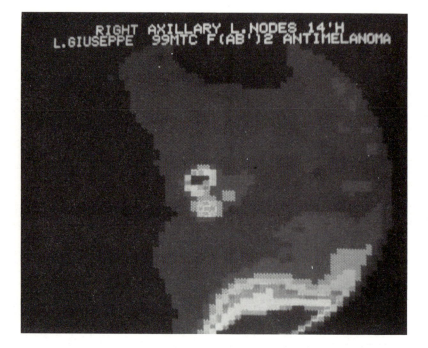

Figure 4 – Right axillary lymph nodes imaged after injection
of the 225.28 S anti/melanoma monoclonal F(ab')$_2$

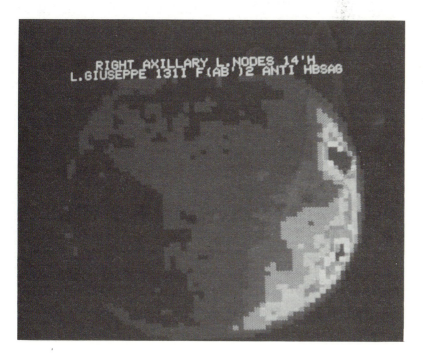

Figure 5 – Same patient of Fig. 4 imaged after injection of
a comparable amount of non specific monoclonal
F(ab')$_2$ (4B5 anti HBsAg).

263

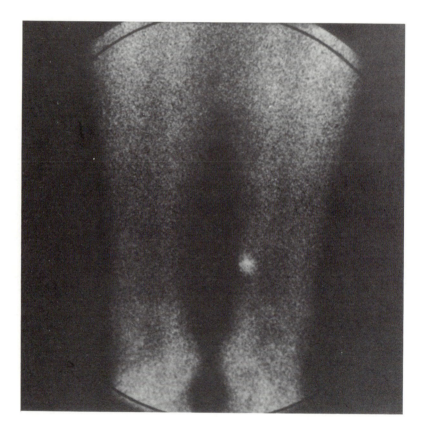

Figure 6 – Unknown subcutaneous lesion 5 mm of diameter
on the left leg.
Scintigram obtained 8 hrs after i.v. injection.

264

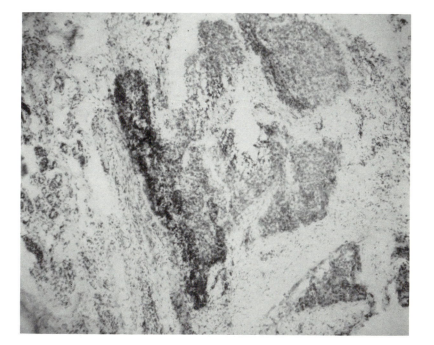

Figure 7 – Unknown subcutaneous lesion 5 mm of diameter
on the left leg.
Immunoperoxidase staining on biopsy material
confirming the lesion.

265

REFERENCES

1. Callegaro L., Deleide G., Dovis M., Cecconato E., Plassio G. and Rosa U.

Purification and labelling of $F(ab')_2$ fragments and their conversion to radiopharmaceuticals.

Proceeding of Saariselka Symposium 10-11 August 1983.

2. Buraggi C., Turrin A., Cascinelli N., Attili A., Bombardieri E. and Gasparini M.

Immunoscintigraphy with melanoma monoclonal antibody.

Proceedings of Saariselka Symposium 10-11 August 1983.

3. Buraggi G.L., Callegaro L., Ferrone S., Turrin A., Cascinelli N., Attili A., Bombardieri E., Mariani G. and Deleide G.

In-vivo immunodiagnosis with radiolabelled anti-melanoma antibodies and $F(ab')_2$ fragments.

Nuclear Medizin: Proceedings of the 21 Int. Ann. Meet. S.N.M.E. Ulm 13-16 Sept. 1983, Ed. Schattauer Verlag, Stuttgart, N.Y., 1984, 713-716.

4. Siccardi A.G.

Antimelanoma monoclonal antibodies in immunoscintigraphy, criteria for a clinical trial of the Italian National Research Council (C.N.R.).

Proceedings of Saariselka Symposium 10-11 August 1983.

Immunodetection of Human Melanoma Metastases by means of F(AB')2 Fragments of Monoclonal Antibodies: The Usefulness of Digital Images.

Masi R.[1], Pesciullesi E.[1], Ferri P.[1], Voegelin M.R.[2], Paladini S.[1], Valecchi C.[3], and Giannotti B[3].

1. Nuclear Medicine Unit, U.S.L. 10/D, Florence (Italy).
2. Nuclear Medicine and Medical Physics Institute, University of Florence.
3. 2nd Dermatology Clinic, University of Florence.

Monoclonal antibodies against melanoma associated antigens (MAA) have been developed and labelled for "in-vivo" immunodetection (1,2,3,4). The biodistribution and clearance studies have demonstrated that fragments F(ab')2 and Fab are more suitable for radioimaging than intact IgG (5,6). The immunological specificity of tumour uptake has been demonstrated in animal models and in man (1,2,4). However, a significant non-specific uptake in normal tissues (liver, spleen, bone marrow, kidney) has been observed (2,4,5) to different degrees, according to the procedure of labelling. This is the most important drawback of immunodetection together with other limiting parameters summarized as follows :

– low tumour/non tumour (T/NT) ratio for two dimensional imaging; this may be partially overcome by SPECT (7,8);

– small tumour size: this may be equally overcome by SPECT

(7);

 - interferring background of vascular pools: this may be overcome by cautious subtraction techniques (8);

 - radioactivity released from the tracer : this limit may be reduced with different radiochemical procedures (as labelling with Indium chelates);

 - heterogeneity of antigenic expression even in the same patient : a cocktail of several MoAbs may reduce this false negativity (9).

The demonstrated faster clearance of F(ab')2 from normal tissues than from tumoural lesions (10,11) and the observation that the absolute value to tumour uptake remains almost stable during the time interval suitable for imaging suggests that contrast may be improved by means of late time interval imaging. For this purpose a radiotracer with a physical half-life longer than its biological half-life must be used.

In the present study ^{111}I-F(ab')2 anti-melanoma were employed. The different C/t function in normal and neoplastic tissues was evaluated as a possible tool for a contrast enhancement technique without the inaccuracies of pair-labelling subtraction techniques.

METHODS

F(ab')2 were prepared from monoclonal antibody 225.28S to HMW-MAA obtained by Ferrone S. (1) and labelled with ^{111}In-chelates (Sorin Biomedica) at a specific activity of 30-50 mCi/mg.

The tracer, purified and controlled at the time of production, was controlled again by Sephadex G 200 gel filtration before injection and in the patients sera at various time intervals (Fig.1).

20 Patients with widespread melanoma (stage IIIB, IIIAb, IV) were selected for the study after their informed consent. Baseline laboratory tests were performed before and after the completion of immunoscintigraphy. Patients received 2-3 mCi (92.5-111 MBq) of In-111 bound to 0.07-0.08 mg of F(ab')2.

The studies were performed with a LFOV scintillation camera interfaced to a data processing system at 48 and 96 hours post injection.

Tc-99m (as albumin or phytate of MDP) was injected, after In-111 image collection at 96 hours, in patients with brain or liver metastases or with lesions near to vascular pools or bone.

Each anatomical region was imaged for 500 kcounts in the same geometrical conditions according to anatomical landmarks.

Digital processing of images was performed through the following steps :

1. Smoothing of non-linear noise. The method employed was based on the identification of the minimum gradient direction in a window 3x3 pixels followed by the substitution of the central pixel with the mean value of pixels located along the direction of minimum gradient.

2. Comparison, through paired images, of the distribution of counting in the two matrices (collected at 48 and 96 hours) after normalization for the total number of counts, with the purpose of evaluating the temporal changes of distribution.

The calculation of local differences was performed after a procedure of matching I_2(96 hours) on I_1(48 hours), shifting I_2 for -h pixels on x axis and for -k pixels on y axis; h and k are the values for which the cross-correlation function R8h,k) is maximal (equation 1):

$$R(h,k) = \sum_{i,j} I_1(i,j) \cdot I_2(i+h,j+k) / \sum \left[I_2(i+h,j+k) \right]^2 \quad (1)$$

This technique, employed for matching of images with equal distribution, needed some adaptations in the present case: I_2 was transformed in I_2 image by means of a procedure of histogram modification to obtain a relative counting rate similar to I_1.

The cross correlation was performed between submatrices with 32x32 dimensions to avoid the shifting out of the 64x64 image.

The pairs of matched and equalized matrices were then submitted to an Ascombe transform: each counting value was transformed according to the equation :

$$I'(i,j) = \langle I(i,j)+3/8 \rangle^{1/2}$$

In I'the noise may be considered additive with a mean value 0 and a variance of 0.25.

This transform avoided more complex methods of comparison between the two images. From the two transformed matrices a new matrix was then generated that displayed the local significance of differences.

Besides the comparison of distribution in paired matrices a comparison inside each matrix was performed : after the selection of a ROl^{on} an invariant area (generally bone marrow), two new matrices were generated representing the percent increase and decrease of counting in each pixel.

RESULTS

Table 1 summarizes the overall results obtained with analogue and digital processed images.

The sensitivity is quite low with analogue images especially for skin and liver lesions, because the former have small dimensions (only 1/13 have a diameter larger than 2 cm) and the latter are hidden in a non specific uptake area.

TABLE 1

OVERALL SENSITIVITY OF ANALOGUE AND DIGITAL PROCESSED IMAGES

Site of lesions	Total	Size of Lesions >2cm	<2cm	Analogic images +ve	-ve	Digital Images +ve	-ve
Skin	13	1	12	1	12	6	7
Liver	11	7	4	2	9	7	4
Lung	4	2	2	0	4	0	4
Brain	5	4	1	4	1	5	0
Adrenal	1	1	0	0	1	0	1
Skeleton	6	3	3	3	3	3	3
Lymphnodes	6	4	2	2	4	6	0
Total	46	22	24	12(25%)	34(74%)	27(59%)	19 (41%)

Table 2, which summarizes the detection rate of lesions wih diameter larger than 2 cm, shows an increase in sensitivity from 26% to 50%. False negative results are still frequent in regions of non specific uptake (liver) or of large vascular pools (lymphnodes of abdomen and pelvis).

However, digital processing of images increases detectiorate to % for all lesions and to 77% for lesions larger than 2 cm.

A lower detection rate is observed for lesions smaller than 2 cm also with digital processed images (Table 3).

Data processing increases the detection rate of tumoral lesions

271

K

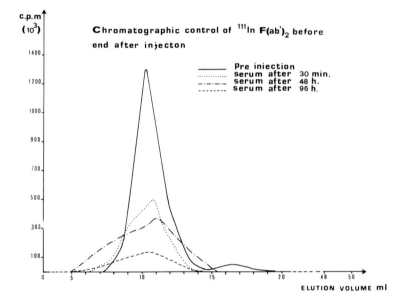

Fig.1 – Gel-filtration of tracer on Sephadex G-200 column before and after adminstration : radiochemical purity and stability are confirmed.

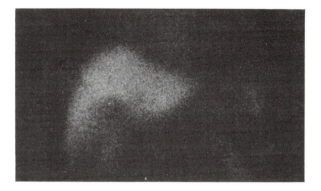

Fig. 2. Analogue scintigraphic image of the upper abdomen 96 hours after injection: liver metastases (six) demonstrated by echography cannot be seen.

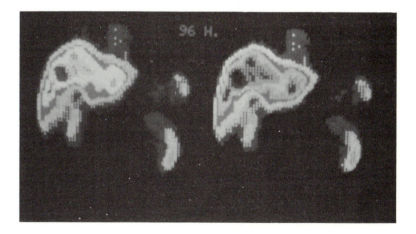

Fig. 3 Digital processed images generated from the comparison between matched images: – on the left the stable or increasing concentration are displayed in red; – on the right the stable or increasing concentrations are displayed in black; the decreasing C/t functions are displayed in other colours (red demonstrates the maximum decrease of concentration). The six tumoral lesions are clearly demonstrated.

of the liver (Fig.2)(7/11 instead of 2/11), lymphnodes (6/6 instead of 2/6) and skin (6/13 instead of 1/13). Fig. 2 and 3 illustrate the image enhancement obtained in a patient with liver matastases.

In our series six metastatic sites (3 lymphnodes, 2 cerebral and 1 bone lesions) were firstly demonstrated by immunoscintigraphy and later confirmed by conventional diagnostic examinations.

TABLE 2

RADIOIMMUNODETECTION OF LESIONS LARGER THAN 2 CM

Sites of lesions	Analogic images	Digital images
Skin	1/1	1/1
Liver	2/7	5/7
Lung	0/2	0/2
Brain	3/4	4/4
Adrenal	0/1	0/1
Skeleton	3/3	3/3
Lymphnodes	2/4	4/4
Total	11/22 (50 %)	17/22 (77 %)

DISCUSSION AND CONCLUSIONS

Our preliminary findings with ^{111}In-F(ab')2 antimelanoma are coherent with the observation of a different clearance rate in tumour and normal tissues (6,10,11,12). The diverging behaviour of C/T function in these sites suggests the opportunity to collect high contrast images at late time intervals, using a radionuclide suitable for this purpose, like in-111 (stability of label and low dose to the patient are other favourable parameters).

TABLE 3

RADIOIMMUNODETECTION OF LESIONS SMALLER THAN 2 CM

Sites of Lesions	Analogic images	Digital images
Skin	0/12	5/12
Liver	0/4	2/4
Lung	0/2	0/2
Brain	0/1	1/1
Skeleton	0/3	0/3
Lymphnodes	0/2	2/2
Total	0/24(0%)	10/24(41%)

This spontaneous contrast enhancement is not sufficient for organs with non specific uptake (liver, spleen, bone marrow). However, the different behaviour of C/t functions may be the basis for a data processing technique able to visualize lesions inside areas of non specific uptake.

In the cases we have investigated this data processing technique increased the detection rate from 50% to 77%, without the artifacts (due to differences in biodistribution energy spectrum, attenuation phenomena) observed with pair labelling subtraction technique.

REFERENCES

1. Wilson B.S., Ruberto G., Ferrone S. Immunochemical characterization of human high molecular weight melanoma

associated antigen identified with monoclonal antibodies. Cancer Immunol. immunother. 14:196 201,1983.

2. Larson M.S., Brown J.P. Wright P.W., Carrasquillo J.A., etal.: Imaging of melanoma with I 131 labelled monoclonal antibodies. J. Nucl. Med. 24:123/129, 1983.

3. Callegaro L., Ferrone S., Plassio G., Dovis M., et al.: Biochemical characterization of monoclonal antibodies and F(ab')2 fragments against human melanoma associated antigen labelled with different radioactive isotopes. J. Nucl. Med. All. Sci. 27:82/83, 1983.

4. Buraggi G.L., Callegaro L., Ferrone S., Turrin A., et al.: In vivo immunodiagnosis with radiolabelled anti melanoma antibodies and F8ab')2 fragments. 21th Intern. Meeting Soc. Nucl. Med. Europe, Ulm W. Germany, 13/16 Sept. 1983.

5. Mariani G., Callegaro L., Mazzuca N., Macchia D., et al.: In vivo distribution of anti human melanoma monoclonal antibodies. In: Protides of the biological fluids Vol.31. Ed. H. Peeters, Pergamon Press, Oxford New York, 1984, Pages 971/976.

6. Burchiel S.W., Khaw B.A., Rhodes B.A., Smith T.W. Haber E.: Immunopharmacokinetics of radiolabelled antibodies and their fragments. In Tumour Imaging. The radiochemical detection of cancer. Eds: Burchiel S.W. and Rhodes B.A., Masson Publ. Inc., Paris, 1982, pages 125/138.

7. Berche D., Mach J.P. Lumbroso J.D., Langlais C., et al.: Tomoscintigraphy for detecting gastrointestinal and medullary thyroid cancers: first clinical results using radiolabelled monoclonal antibodies against carcinoembryonic antigen. Brit. Med. J. 285: 1447/1451, 1982.

8. Deland F.H., Kim E., Simmons G.H., Goldenberg D.M.: Imaging of radiolabelled antibodies for tumour detection. In:

Tumour Imaging. The radiochemical detection of cancer. Eds: Burchiel S.W. and Rhodes B.A., Masson Publ. Inc., Paris, 1982, pages 151/156.

9. Sears H.F., Atkinson B., Mattis J., et al: Phase I clinical trial of monoclonal antibody in treatment of gastrointestinal tumours. Lancet 1 : 762/765, 1982.

10. Larson S.M., Carrasquillo J.A., Krohn K.A., Brown J.P., et al.: Localization of 131 I labelled p97 specific Fab fragments in human melanoma as a basis for radiotherapy. J. Clin. Invest. 72: 1/14, 1983.

11. Herlyn D., Powe J., Alavi A., et al.: Radioimmunodetection of human tumour xenografts by monoclonal antibodies. Cancer Res. 43: 2731/2735, 1983.

12. Chatal J.F., Saccavini J.C., Fumoleau P., Douillard J.Y., et al.: Immunoscintigraphy of colon carcinoma. J. Nucl. Med; 25:307/314, 1983.

The Immunoscintigraphy of Bone Tumours Using an [131] I-Labelled Anti-Osteosarcoma Monoclonal Antibody

Perkins A.C.[1], Armitage N.C.[2], Hardy J.G.[1], Wastie M.L.[3], Pimm M.V.[4] and Hardcastle J.D.[2]

1. Department of Medical Physics.
2. Department of Surgery.
3. Department of Radiology, Nottingham University Hospital.
4. Cancer Research Campaign Laboratories, Nottingham University.

INTRODUCTION

Osteogenic sarcoma is the most common malignant primary tumour of bone. As with most sarcomas tumour spread is invariably via the bloodstream to the lungs and occasionally to other bone sites resulting in a 5 year survival rate of 5–20%. The concurrent development of osteosarcoma in members of the same family implicates genetic or infectious factors. In addition a high incidence of anti-osteosarcoma antibodies has been found in the sera of patients and their close associates.

In 1895 Hericourt and Richet (1) raised antisera against human osteosarcom which was found to be effective against a fibrosarcom of the chest wall and a stomach cancer. A range of monoclonal antibodies which react with osteosarcoma cells has been developed by the Cancer Research Campaign Laboratories at Nottingham University (2). One of these antibodies designated 7911/36 was found to localise in human osteosarcoma xenografts maintained in immunodeprived mice. Labelling of the antibody with ^{131}I enabled detection of the uptake at the xenograft site (3) . These findings prompted the clinical study of the in vivo localisation of this antibody in a patient with osteosarcoma of the right knee (4). In the present study the same antibody has been used in a series of patients with suspected malignant primary bone tumours.

PATIENTS AND METHODS

Fourteen patients with an age range of 5–65 years were included in the study. Each patient presented with a high suspicion of a malignant bone tumour and radiographs and ^{99m}Tc-MDP bone images were obtained prior to the antibody study.

The antibody was radiolabelled using ^{131}I as described previously (3). A subcutaneous injection of the antibody was administered to each patient to test for anaphylaxis, followed 15 minutes later by an intravenous dose containing 200 ug antibody labelled with 70 MBq ^{131}I, except in the case of the 5 year old child who received a 30 MBq dose. Thyroid uptake of any unbound radioiodide was blocked by oral administration of potassium iodide. Patients were imaged 48 hours after antibody administration using a large field of view gamma camera fitted with a high energy collimator (400 keV maX.). Data were stored by computer in a 64x64 matrix. Background subtraction was carried out using ^{99m}Tc-labelled red blood cells and sodium pertechnetate and additional views were acquired after administration of ^{113m}In-indium chloride to label the blood transferrin. Subtraction of the technetium images from the iodine images resulted in large artefacts outside the patient which were particularly noticeable on images of the limbs. A computer threshold subtraction of the ^{131}I view before ^{99m}Tc subtraction and the use of ^{113m}In subtraction resulted in a reduction of artefacts (5).

The patient diagnosis was confirmed by biopsy in each case and the final results were compared with radiographs and the ^{99m}Tc MDP bone images.

Table 1. PRIMARY BONE TUMOURS
(ANTI-OSTEOSARCOMA MONOCLONAL ANTIBODY)

PATIENT SEX AGE	HISTOLOGY	SITE	^{131} IMAGE	BLOOD POOL	SUBTRACTION
F 16	Osteosarcoma	femur	+	+	+
M 26	Osteosarcoma	ileum	+	+	+
F 16	Osteosarcoma	tibia	+	+	+
F 24	Parosteal osteosarcoma	tibia	+	−	+
M 33	Ewings sarcoma	femur	+	+	+
F 24	benign osteoblastoma	tibia	+	−	+
M 22	Osteochondroma	femur	+	+	+
F 53	Giant cell tumour	tibia	+	+	−
M 49	histiocytic sarcoma	radius/ ulna	−	−	−

Patient details and imaging results of nine patients with primary bone tumours.

RESULTS

Positive localisation of labelled antibody was seen in seven out of the nine patients who were found to have primary bone tumours, four of which were osteosarcomas. Results of histology and imaging are given in Table 1. In eight patients increased activity could be seen at the tumour site on the ^{131}I images before background subtraction. However in six cases the blood pool images also showed greater activity, therefore the subtracted images were used to assess positive tumour uptake of antibody. Positive uptake in a 26 year old male with osteosarcoma of the right ileum is shown in Fig. 1. The imaging results and histology for the remaining five patients are given in Table 2. Positive uptake was identified in 2 patients with osteomyelitis, the remaining two patients with stress fractures and one with a bone cyst failed to show concentration of the labelled antibody. Thirteen patients had ^{99m}Tc-MDP bone imaging which in each case showed increased uptake at the site of the lesion.

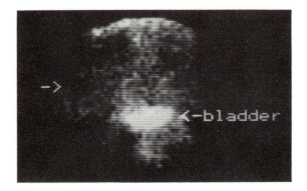

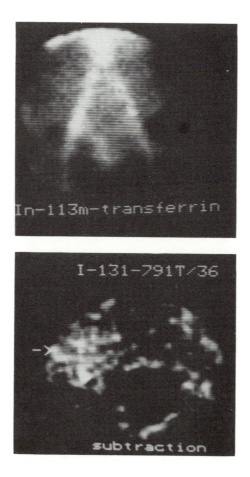

Figure 1. Gamma scintigraphy of a patient with osteosarcoma of the right ileum. Anterior views of the pelvis showing 131-I -79IT/36 image. ^{113m}In-transferrin blood pool image and subtracted image after masking the bladder by computer (arrow indicates tumour site).

BONE TUMOURS

TABLE 2. OTHER BONE LESIONS

PATIENT Sex Age	HISTOLOGY	SITE	^{131}I-IMAGE	BLOOD POOL-SUBTRACTION	
M 50	osteomyelitis	tibia	+	+	+
F 56	osteomyelitis	femur	+	–	+
F 17	stress	fibula	–	–	–
F 5	stress	tibia	+	+	–
F 24	bone cyst	femur	–	–	–

Patient details and imaging results of five patients with other bone lesions

DISCUSSION

The present study has demonstrated increased uptake of monoclonal antibody 791T/36 in a high proportion of the primary bone tumours studied in this group of patients. In one patient with a histiocytic sarcoma who failed to show uptake of the radiolabelled antibody the tumour was found to be microscopic in size and it is doubtful whether any uptake would be expected to be visualised by this technique. The uptake of the antibody in two patients with osteomyelitis suggests that other non-malignant lesions are capable of concentrating the antibody.

Blood pool subtraction was found to be necessary with this ^{131}I preparation to exclude the vascular component when assessing positive tumour localisation of antibody. The 791T/36 antibody appeared to be more selective than ^{99m}Tc-MDP bone imaging and was taken up more avidly by the more aggressive malignant tumours. However the use of this technique for diagnosis is limited when compared to other diagnostic modalities and it may be that the antibody is more appopriate for targetting therapeutic agents. The 791T/36 antibody has been conjugated to vindesine to produce a drug-antibody conjugate which was preferentially cytotoxic for osteosarcoma cells (6). The present study has shown uptake of the monoclonal antibody 791T/36 in a range of primary bone lesions and gives support to the potential use of immune mediated therapy.

REFERENCES

(1) Hericourt,J.& Richet,C. (1895) De la selatherapie dans le treatment du cancer.

Comptes Rendus hebdomadaire des sceances de l'academie des

sciences 121.567–569.

(2) Embledon,M.J. et al (1981) Anti-tumour reactions of monoclonal antibody against a human osteogenic sarcoma cell line.

Br.J.Canc. 43. 582–587.

(3) Pimm,M.V. et al (1982) In vivo localisation of anti-osteogenic sarcoma 791T monoclonal antibody in osteogenic sarcoma xenografts.

Int.J.Canc.30.75–85.

(4) Farrands,P.A. et al (1983) Localisation of human osteosarcoma by antitumour monoclonal antibody.

J.Bone & Joint Surg.65B .638–640.

(5) Perkins,A.C. et al (1984) Physical approach for the reduction of dual radionuclide image subtraction artefacts in immunoscintigraphy.

Nuc.Med.Comm.5.501–512.

(6) Embleton,M.J. et al (1983) Selective cytotoxicity against human tumour cells by a vindesine monoclonal antibody conjugate.

Br.J.Canc.46.43–49.

Immunoscintigraphy of Metastasizing Prostatic Carcinoma with Prostatic Acid Phosphatase-specific Antibodies

Vihko P., Heikkila J, Kontturi M., Lukkarinen O., Wahlberg L. and Vihko R.

Department of Clinical Chemistry and Department of Surgery, University of Oulu, SF–90220 Oulu, Finland.

INTRODUCTION

We have previously shown that ^{99m}Tc- or ^{111}In-labelled DTPA (diethylene triamine penta-acetic acid) –derivatives of polyclonal antibodies or their Fab fragments against a prostatic secretory protein, acid phosphatase, can be used to reveal metastases of prostatic carcinoma (1,2). Specifically, bone metastases were also detected. Lee et al. (3) used a monoclonal antiprostatic acid phosphatase antibody and an ^{125}I-label in studies on human prostate tumour xenografted in nude mice, and Goldenberg et al (4) used an ^{131}I-labelled rabbit antibody against prostatic acid phosphatase in two patients with prostatic cancer. In these patients, the bone metastases present were not revealed by the technique used.

We have extended our studies to incorporate 10 patients in addition to the 7 previously reported (1,2). Our first results on the use of F8ab)$_2$ fragments of polyclonal antibodies, and of monoclonal antibody are also reported here.

MATERIALS AND METHODS

PATIENTS

Seventeen patients with prostatic cancer were investigated. Of these 15 had $T_{3-4}N_{x-1}M_1$, one had $T_3N_xm_0$, and one had $T_0N_xm_0$ disease (5). Fourteen patients have been studied using a ^{99m}Tc-label. In 13 patients, polyclonal antibodies were used: in 10 cases the whole antibody, in 2 cases the $F(ab)_2$ fragment, and in one case, the Fab fragment. One experiment was performed using a monoclonal antibody. One patient, first studied with the use of a whole specific ^{99m}Tc-labelled antibody, was later studied using a non-specific rabbit IgG preparation, treated and labelled identically to the specific antibody.

An ^{111}In-label has been used in 3 patients. Two experiments have been carried out using polyclonal antibodies and one with monoclonal antibodies.

Prior to injection, the patients were checked for hypersensitivity using the DTPA-derivative, before labelling with the radionuclide, using the Mantoux technique.

METHODS

The main human prostatic acid phosphatase, purified to homogeneity (6), was used to raise antibodies in rabbits. The same antigen was used in the preparation of monoclonal antibodies, to be described separately (Vihko P. et al., manuscript in preparation). The antibodies were purified by affinity chromatography using immobilized PAP, and Fab and $F(ab)_2$ fragments were purified on protein A Sepharose following papain or pepsin digestion, respectively. DTPA-derivatives of the antibodies and their fragments were prepared (8) and labelled with ^{99m}Tc (9) or ^{111}In (10). The labelled antibodies and their Fab fragments; were sterile filtered and diluted with physiological saline prior to injection. A rota-Camera ZLC 75 (Siemens), equipped with a PDP 11/34 computer (Gamma-11 system) and Micro Dot imager was used for recordings at timed intervals up to 2-3 days. No image processing or subtraction techniques were used. Bone scanning was performed using ^{99m}Tc-DPD (3,3-diphosphono-1,2-propanedicarbonic acid).

RESULTS

POLYCLONAL ANTIBODIES AND THEIR FRAGMENTS

The amounts of whole antibodies injected have varied between 135 and 500 ug, those of F(ab)$_2$ have been 200 ug in both cases studied, and that of Fab, 50 ug in the single case studied. The dose of radioactivity (^{99m}Tc-label) has been 2-9 mCi in the case of whole polyclonal antibodies, 19 mCi when the F(ab)$_2$ fragments have been used and 4 mCi in the case of the Fab fragments. In the two instances in which polyclonal antibodies were labelled with ^{111}In, the doses of radioactivity were 0.7 and 2.8 mCi, respectively.

The results obtained with whole polyclonal antibodies and the two labels, ^{99m}Tc and ^{111}In, are shown in Figs. 1 and 2, respectively. In Fig. 1 it can be seen that the radioactivity injected was first detected in the blood circulation, and then it rapidly appeared in the liver and kidneys. Metastases became visible more slowly and when ^{99m}Tc-label is used, the maximum resolution of metastases was seen at approximately 24 h following injection. Fig. 1 also shows that the non-specific rabbit IgG, labelled with ^{99m}Tc, did not become incorporated in the metastatic lesions.

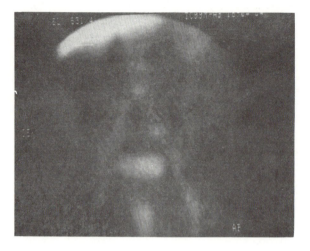

Figure 1 (left)

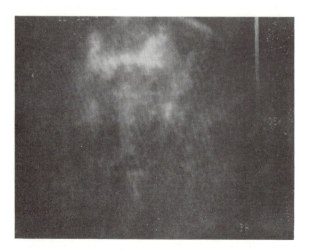

Figure 1 (middle)

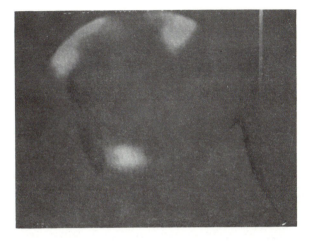

Figure 1 (right)

Left and middle panels: Immunoscintigraphy using
^{99m}Tc-labelled (7 mCi) polyclonal affinity-purified antibodies (170 ug) against human prostate-specific acid phosphatase. Left: 6 h; middle: 24 following i.v. injection. Right panel: Immunoscintigraphy of the same patient using ^{99m}Tc-labelled (8 mCi) polyclonal non-specific rabbit IgG (200 ug). 24 h following injection.

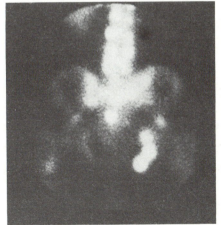

Figure 2 (left)

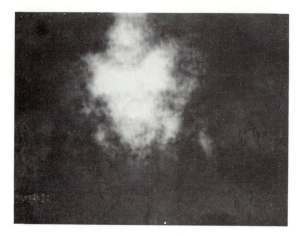

Figure 2 (right)

Left panel: Bone scanning with ^{99m}Tc-DPD in a patient with advanced prostatic cancer. Right panel: Immunoscintigraphy of the same patient using ^{111}In-labelled (0.7 mCi) polyclonal affinity-purified antibodies (250 ug) against human prostate-specific acid phosphatase. 48 h following injection.

Fig. 2 shows the incorporation of whole polyclonal antibody labelled with ^{111}In into the large pelvic metastases also detected in conventional bone scanning. Irrespective of the antibody or its fragment, or the label used, there has been excellent correlation between the findings in immunoscintigraphy and bone scanning. Our limited experience with ^{111}In suggests that the radioactivity may be efficiently recorded up to at least 48 h following injection. So far, the information obtained with the use of Fab or F(ab)$_2$ fragments is comparable to that with polyclonal antibodies.

MONOCLONAL ANTIBODIES

Two experiments have been performed using whole antibodies, one with a ^{99m}Tc- and the other with an ^{111}In-label. One patient with $T_3N_xM_0$-disease was studied using monoclonal antibodies (210 ug) and an ^{111}In-label (3.7 mCi). After 48 h, para-aortic lymnphnode metastases could be seen (Fig. 3).

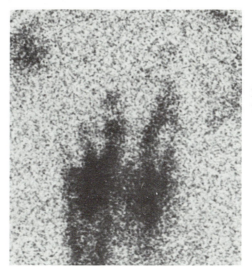

Figure 3.
Immunoscintigraphy using ^{111}In-labelled (3.7 mCi) monoclonal affinity-purified antibodies (210 ug) against human prostate–specific acid phosphatase. Lymphnode metastases at the L3-region. 48 h following injection.

This finding was later confirmed by CT-lymphography which clearly showed lymphnode metastases at the L3-level on the left side. The other patient, with $T_0N_xM_0$-disease, was investigated using monoclonal antibodies (500 ug) and a ^{99m}Tc-label (7 mCi). After 24 h, no metastases were detected.

DISCUSSION

The present study extends our previous ones (1,2) by showing that, in addition to whole polyclonal antibodies and their Fab fragments, $F(ab)_2$ fragments of polyclonal antibodies, and monoclonal antibodies against human prostate-specific acid phosphatase can be used for visualization of metastases of prostatic cancer. We have used DTPA-derivatives of the protein moieties and ^{99m}Tc or ^{111}In as the label, and both labels seem suitable for the purpose.

The present results also show that in one patient with advanced prostatic cancer, the incorporation of radioactivity into metastatic tissue following injection of ^{99m}Tc-labelled polyclonal specific antibodies is a property not shared by non-specific rabbit IgG. Despite the fact that the precise site of the radioactivity in the carcinoma tissue is not known at present, this finding strongly suggests that specific processes are involved in the incorporation of radioactivity into prostatic cancer tissue. This finding encourages extension of these studies to preoperative staging of patients with prostatic cancer.

REFERENCES

1. Vihko P., Heikkila J., Kontturi M., Wahlberg L., Vihko R. Radioimaging of the prostate and metastases of prostatic carcinoma with ^{99m}Tc-labelled prostatic acid phosphatase-specific antibodies and their Fab fragments.
Ann. Clin. Res. 1984; 16: 51-2.

2. Vihko P., Heikkila J., Kontturi M., Lukkarinen O., Wahlberg L., Vihko R. Radioimaging of prostatic carcinoma with prostatic acid phosphatase-specific polyclonal antibodies. Protides of the Biological Fluids, Proceedings 1984, in press.

3. Lee C.L., Kawinski E., Leong S.S. Horosziewicz J.S. Murphy G.P., Chu T.M. Radioimmunodetection and immunochemotherapy of xenografted human prostatic tumour using monoclonal antibody. Fed. Proc. 1983; 42:682 (abstract 2284).

4. Goldenberg D.M., Deland F.H., Bennett S.J., Primus F.J., Nelson M.G., Flanigan R.C. McRoberts J.W. Bruce A.W., Mahan D.E. radioimmunodetection of prostatic cancer. In vivo use of radioactive antibodies against prostatic acid phosphatase for diagnosis and detection of prostatic cancer by nuclear imaging. J. Am. Med. Ass. 1983; 250:630-5.

5. Harmer M.H. Prostate. In: TNM classification of malignant tumours. Geneva: International Union Against Cancer, 178: 118-21.

6. Vihko P., Kontturi M., Korhonen L.K. Purification of human prostatic acid phosphatase by affinity chromatography and isoelectric focusing . Part I. Clin. Chem. 1978; 24: 466-70.

7. Vihko P., Sajanti E., Janne O., Peltonen L., Vihko R. Serum prostate-specific acid phosphatase: development and validation of a specific radioimmunoassay. Clin. Chem. 178; 24:1915-9.

8. Krejcarek G.E. Tucker K.L. Covalent attachment of chelating groups to macromolecules. Biochem. Biophys. Res. Comm. 1977; 77:581-5.

9. Khaw B.A., Strauss H.W., Carvalho A., Locke E., Gold H.K., Haber E. Technetium-99m labelling of antibodies to cardiac myosin Fab and to human fibrinogen. J. Nucl. Med. 1982; 23: 1011-9.

10. Fairweather D.S., Bradwell A.R., Dykes P.W., Vaughan A.T., Watson-James S.F., Chandler S., Improved tumour localization using indium-111 labelled antibodies. Br. Med. J. 1983; 287:167-70.

Evaluation of the Immunoscintigraphy of Gynaecological Tumours

A.C. PERKINS [1], J.G. HARDY [1], E.M. SYMONDS [2], M.L. WASTIE [3] AND M.V. PIMM [4]

1. Department of Medical Physics,

2. Department of Obstetrics and Gynaecology,

3. Department of Radiology, Nottingham University Hospital,

4. Cancer Research Campaign Laboratories, Nottingham University.

INTRODUCTION

The use of radiolabelled antitumour antibodies for the detection of malignancies has increased considerably over the past few years. Much attention is being placed on the use of monclonal antibodies in attempts to improve the specificity of localisation. The pattern of antigen expression defined by monoclonal antibodies is such that a single antibody type can be used to image a variety of malignancies. Monoclonal antibodies including those to carcinoembryonic antigen and milk fat globule have been shown previously to localise in ovarian carcinoma (1)(2). The antibody 791T/36 originally prepared against human osteogenic sarcoma cells, has been used successfully to localise in primary osteogenic sarcoma (3) in primary and secondary colorectal carcinoma (4) and in tumours of the breast (5). In the present study the same antibody radiolabelled with ^{131}I has been used in the investigation of patients with gynaecological tumours in order to evaluate the clinical role of the technique.

PATIENTS AND METHODS

Patients in the present study comprised of 12 with ovarian tumours, four with carcinoma of the cervix and two with carcinoma of the body of the uterus. Of the 12 patients with carcinoma of the ovary, eight were imaged prior to surgery which was being performed as a second look procedure for recurrent disease. Six patients had adenocarcinoma of the ovary and a seventh patient had a tumour which was initially considered to be a benign mucinous cystadenoma but was subsequently considered malignant. Two patients had recurrent granulosa cell carcinomas and one had a squamous cell carcinoma arising in a dermoid cyst. One patient was found to have a primary mucous secreting adenocarcinoma not involving the pelvic organs and a further patient had a benign serous cyst in an ovarian remnant following pelvic clearance. Three patients had proven carcinoma of the cervix and a further patient with clinical suspicion of carcinoma of the cervix was found to be normal at surgery. One patient had and endometrial adenocarcinoma of the body of the uterus and a further patient had a benign cellular leiomyoma of the uterus.

To block thyroid uptake of free iodide patients were given oral potassium iodide throughout the study. A 1 ml subcutaneous test dose was given before injection of the antibody to test for anaphylaxis and subsequently 10 ml of solution containing 200 ug of antibody labelled with 70 MBq ^{131}I was injected into the antecubital vein of the patient's right arm. Patients were imaged between 18h and 48h after administration of the antibody. Anterior and posterior images of the abdomen and pelvic regions were acquired using a gamma camera having a 40 cm field of view fitted with a high energy collimator and data were stored by computer. ^{99m}Tc-labelled erythrocytes and free pertechnetate were used to simulate the distribution of the labelled antibody in circulation. After acquisition of the second image and thresholding of the ^{131}I view background subtraction was carried out as described by (6).

RESULTS

Uptake of labelled antibody was demonstrated in 16 out of the 18 patients investigated. Results are given in Table 1. In five patients with ovarian tumours abnormal uptake could be determined on the ^{131}I images alone, however as this may have been due to the volume of circulating activity within highly vascular lesions subtraction of the blood pool was performed in all patient studies. An example of a patient with a recurrent ovarian carcinoma is given in Figure 1.

In all cases with malignant disease positive uptake of labelled antibody was identified irrespective of the type of malignancy. One patient with ovarian cystadenocarcinoma was re-investigated following radiotherapy and the sites of uptake were markedly reduced in size in the second study, in keeping with her clinical improvement. Another patient who was considered to have a benign mucinous cytadenoma showed pelvic uptake superior to the bladder. Review of the histology lead to a revised diagnosis of mucinous cystadenocarcinoma. No abnormal uptake was demonstrated in a patient with a benign serous cystadenoma and in one patient who was thought to have carcinoma of the cervix but had a normal pelvis at surgery. In all the patients concentration of radioiodine was observed in the spleen and in the urine.

DISCUSSION

The monoclonal antibody 791T/36 has been used to image malignancies of the ovary, cervix and uterus with a high degree of accuracy. No localisation was demonstrated in one patient with a

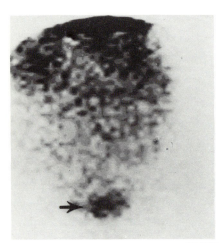

A

B

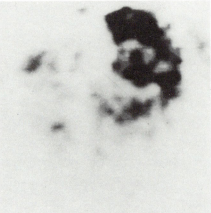

Figure 1

Anterior images of the pelvis of a patient with recurrent granulosa cell carcinoma of the ovary. a) ^{131}I-labelled antibody distribution (arrow indicates iodide in the bladder) b) region of tumour uptake shown after ^{99m}Tc-background subtraction.

300

Case No.

Ovary

1 - 6	Adenocarcinoma	+ve
7	Primary mucous secreting adenocarcinoma (? pancreas)	+ve
8 - 9	Recurrent granulosa cell carcinoma	+ve
10	Squamous cell carcinoma in dermoid cyst	+ve
11	Mucous cystadenocarcinoma	+ve
12	Benign serous cyst in ovarian remnant	+ve

Cervix

13	Recurrent carcinoma of cervix	+ve
14	" " "	+ve
15	" " "	+ve
16	Normal pelvis at surgery	−ve

Uterus

| 17 | Adenocarcinoma of endometrium | +ve |
| 18 | Benign cellular leiomyoma | +ve |

Table 1. Results of 18 patients with Gynaeocological Tumours Imaged with ^{131}I-791T/36.

benign ovarian mass and another patient who was subsequently found to be normal at surgery. Uptake was seen however in a benign cellular leiomyoma of the uterus. The extent of tumour involvement from the images has been used to aid radiotherapy treatment planning in one patient and repeat investigation provided a useful follow-up. However, the accuracy of spatial measurement from images after background subtraction is questionable. Repeat investigations have been performed in four further patients in this study and has proved useful in the assessment of recurrent disease. The high degree of reliability in imaging malignant disease indicates that the technique probably offers the greatest clinical value in the assessment of tumour recurrence and offers an alternative to second-look surgical procedures with their accompanying morbidity in the older age group patients. However, antibody response against mouse immunoglobulin has been detected in patients sera. Using sephacryl S-300 gel-filtration, high molecular weight complexes of antibody have been identified in patient serum after repeated injection of 791T/36 antibody. This could represent one of the major limitations of what appears to be the most promising application of immunoscintigraphy in patients with gynaecological cancer.

REFERENCES

1) Armitage, N.C., Perkins, A.C. Pimm, M.V., Farrands, P.A., Baldwin, R.W. and Hardcastle, J.D. 1984. The localisation of an anti-tumour monoclonal antibody (791T/36) in gastrointestinal tumours. Br. J. Surg. 71: 407–412.

2) Epenetos, A.A., Mather, S., Granowska, M., Nimmon, C.C., Hawkins, L.R., Britton, K.E., Shepherd, J., Taylor-Papadimitriou, J., Durbin, H., Malpas, J.S. and Bodmer, W.F. 1982. Targetting of iodine-123-labelled tumour associated monoclonal antibodies to ovarian, breast and gastrointestinal tumours. Lancet 2: 999–1004.

3) Farrands, P.A., Perkins, A.C., Sully, L., Hopkins, J.S., Pimm, M.V., Baldwin, R.W. and Hardcastle, J.D. 1983. Localisation of

human osteosarcoma by anti-tumour monoclonal antibody. J. Bone & Joint Surg. 65-B: 638-640.

4) Mach,J.P., Buchegger, F., Forni, M., Ritschard, J., Berche, C., Lumbroso, J.D.., Schreyer, M., Giraroet, C., Accolla, R.S. and Carrel, S. 1981. Use of radiolabelled monoclonal anti-CEA antibodies for the detection of human carcinomas by external photoscanning and tomoscintigraphy. Immunol. Today 2: 239-249.

5) Perkins, A.C., Whalley, D.R. and Hardy, J.G. 1984. Physical approach for the reduction of dual radionuclide image subtraction artefacts in immunoscintigraphy. Nucl. Med. Comm. 5: 501-512.

6) Williams, M.R., Perkins, A.C., Campbell, F.C., Pimm, M.V., Hardy, J.G., Wastie, M.L., Blamey, R.W. and Baldwin, R.W. 1984. The use of monoclonal antibody 791T/36 in the immunoscintigraphy of primary and metastatic carcinoma of the breast. Clinical Oncology. In press.

L

Stability of In-111 Labelled DTPA Modified Proteins: Human Albumin, Bovine Fibrinogen and Monoclonal Antibody against Human Milk Fat Globule Antigen

Goedemans W.Th 1), de Jong M.M.Th 1), van Dulmen A.A. 1)
Haisma H.H. 2), Hilkens J. 2)

1) Mallinckrodt Diagnostica Holland B.V., Petten,
The Netherlands.
2) The Netherlands Cancer Institute, Amsterdam,
The Netherlands.

INTRODUCTION

During the past years alternative procedures to the direct radioiodination technique have been suggested in order to decrease the damage to the proteins occurring during the labelling process and to eliminate the fact of deiodination in the body after in vivo application of radiolabelled proteins. The direct metal labelling of biologically active proteins is difficult, because of the lack of specific metal binding receptors.

A solution to this problem is to attach to protein chelating agents capable of providing a high stability binding site. In choosing the coupling reaction two prerequisites have to be considered.

1) The chelon must attach in such a way, that the product retains its biological properties.

305

2) The chosen metal ion(s) must form bonds with the conjugate chelates which dissociate very slowly or not at all under in vitro and in vivo conditions.

The first approach to covalently coupling chelating groups to macromolecules was reported by Benisek and Richards (1968), who reacted lysozyme with methyl picolinimidate to produce a bidentate chelating site. In 1974 Sundberg et al (1974) utilized a bifunctional analog of EDTA (ethylenediamine tetraacetic acid) to create specific metal chelating sites on macromolecules.

Their technique used a phenyl EDTA molecule which could be derivatized in the paraposition of the aromatic ring. Specifically 1-(p-benzenediazonium) EDTA was synthesized and coupled to several proteins.

Krejcarek and Tucker (1977) described a procedure, which attaches the polyaminocarboxylate chelating agent DTPA (diethylenetriamine penta acetic acid) to a protein as human serum albumin. This procedure was also followed by Khaw et al (1980) who coupled DTPA to Fab fragments of antimyosine antibodies. Other candidates used as interchelate between radiometal and protein are: nitrilotriacetic acid (NTA) (Gokce et al 1982), transferrin (Wolf et al 1982), dithiosemicarbazone (Yokoyama et al 1982 and 1983), deferoxamine (Janoki et al 1982 and 1983, Yokoyama et al 1982, Ohmomo et al 1982).

A simple and efficient method of covalently coupling DTPA to proteins by using the bicyclic anhydride of DTPA was developed by Hnatowich et al (1982) for albumin, by Layne et al (1982) for fibronogen and by Hnatowich et al (1983) for immunoglobulin G antibodies.

Successful imaging of tumours using labelled monoclonal

antibody will largely depend on the integrity of the labelled antibody and the stability of the bond between protein and radionuclide. If labelled monoclonal antibody for example is injected into the animal it can last 24 hours or more before the relatively slow clearance has enabled imaging.

During this period and if possible for longer the radionuclide has to stay connected to the protein and the biological activity must not disappear. We approached this situation in vitro by stability testing at $38-40^{\circ}$ and by assessing at intervals the specific activity of the labelled protein. Proteins of choice were bovine fibrinogen, human albumin (used as a model proteins in our labelling experiments) and monoclonal antibody against human milkfat globule antigen (Hilkens et al 1983) which was supplied by the Anthonie van Leeuwenhoekhuis. We coupled DTPA to the protein using the bicyclic DTPA anhydride method of Layne et al (1982) and Hnatowich et al (1983) and labelled it with In-111 using tris acetate buffered In-111 oxinate pH 7 (Goedemans 1981). We tested sucrose and hydroxyethyl starch as possible stabilizing agents.

MATERIALS AND METHODS

Source of some essential chemicals and biochemicals.
Bovine Fibrinogen, Povite (Poviet Producten N.V.) Amsterdam, The Netherlands.
Buminate 25 %, Normal serum Albumin (Human) Hyland Therapeutics, Division Travenol Laboratories Inc.
DTPA diethylene triamine penta acetic acid, J.T.Baker Chemicals B.V., Deventer, The Netherlands
Monoclonal antibody 115 D8 (m.c.a.), Anthonie van

Leeuwenhoekhuis, Amsterdam, The Netherlands.
Sephadex G50 fine, Pharmacia Uppsala, Sweden.
In-111 oxinate, Mallinckrodt Diagnostica Holland B.V.,
Petten, The Netherlands.
Iron-59 as chloride in 0.1 M HCl 3-20 mCi/mg Fe TRC
Amersham U.K. hydroxyethyl starch (h.e.s.), trade name
Plasmasteril, Fresenius, Bad Homburg, W. Germany.

protein labelling

The bicyclic DTPA anhydride, prepared by a simple one-step
synthesis, according to Eckelman (1975), was added as the solid to
the solid or the solid to the liquid protein.

DTPA was covalently coupled to protein via the bicyclic
anhydride of DTPA. DTPA continues to form stable chelates
despite the loss of one carboxyl group in the formation of the
amide bond.

Coupling was completed in minutes at room temperature. DTPA
forms among the strongest 1:1 chelates known for a large number
of metals such as In^{3+} or Ga^{3+}.

Protein was dissolved in PBS in different quantities depending
on the ratio DTPA : Protein to be achieved. For albumin this
ratio was 10:1, for fibrinogen 50:1 and for m.c.a. 22:1. These were
calculated ratios based on the amount of bicyclic DTPA anhydride
and protein offered. Due to some hydrolysis of the anhydride
during the coupling reactions the ratios obtained in practice will
be lower.

The protein solution was added to be dried DTPA anhydride
and incubated for 5 minutes at room temperature under magnetic
stirring. The reaction mixture was purified by gel chromatography

(sephadex G 50 column 15 cm) separating DTPA-protein from free DTPA. This DTPA-protein was ready for labelling with In-111l oxinate. This labelling was simply accomplished by adding the desired amount of In-111 oxinate buffered at pH7. In-111 exchanged from the oxine to the DTPA chelate on the protein. (Goedemans, to be published).

Free In-111 was removed from the protein by means of G50 sephadex gel chromatography.

Stability testing

The In-111 DTPA coupled protein was sterilized by Millex filter units and divided into 1 ml samples These 1 ml samples containing ca 0.3 mg protein were stored at $40^{\circ}C$ during 1,4 or 7 days (115 D8). Labelled fibrinogen samples were stored 1,2 or 5 days at $38^{\circ}C$. In some cases In-111 labelled proteins were incubated in a 4.5% sucrose (in PBS) solution or hydroxyethyl starch 3% (in PBS) pH 7.4. Stability of the labelled protein was tested by subjecting the stored samples to gel chromatography (Sephadex G50) in order to separate · any loose indium from the protein-DTPA and to check any protein decomposition. Specific activities were assessed by relating protein amount and radioactivity of the collected fractions. The biological activity of monoclonal antibody 115 D8 after storage at $40^{\circ}C$ for 7 days was determined by means of Elisa testing.

Stability testing of albumin-DTPA-In-111 in the presence of Fe-59

Before incubation with albumin-DTPA-In-111, Fe-59 was

309

complexed to citrate 0.13 M pH 7.8.

Albumin-DTPA-In-111 was first incubated with 0.1 mg non radioactive Fe^{+++} as citrate (0.13 M) for 20 minutes at room temperature to occupy empty DTPA sites.

The Albumin-DTPA-In-111 was incubated with 5uCi Fe-59 citrate for 65 hours at $40^{\circ}C$, so that eventual coupling of Fe-59 to protein would be the result of ion exchange.

The albumin blank was treated with In-111 oxinate and after removing of free In-111 with 0.1 mg Fe^{+++} as citrate (0.13 M) for 20 minutes, then with 5uCi Fe-59 in the same way.

There was also an albumin-DTPA-In-111 control not treated with Fe-59 but also incubated for 65 hours at $40^{\circ}C$.

After incubation all In-111 and Fe-59 treated samples were subjected to Sephadex G50 gel chromatography collecting samples of 1.5 ml in which absorbance at 280 nm, In-111 and Fe-59 radioactivity were measured.

Radioactivity measurement being done on a Ge-Li scintillation detector for proper discrimination of the two isotopes.

RESULTS

Stability of bovine fibrinogen-DTPA labelled with
In-111 oxinate

Fibrinogen-DTPA In-111 elution profiles (chromatograph on sephadex G50 fine) are presented in Fig.1. The upper part shows the profiles if PBS is used as solvent. The lower part the profiles if 4.5% sucrose in PBS is used as solvent. It is clear that indium labelled fibrinogen is quite stable under the circumstances studied and it does not matter whether or not sucrose is used as stabilizing agent.

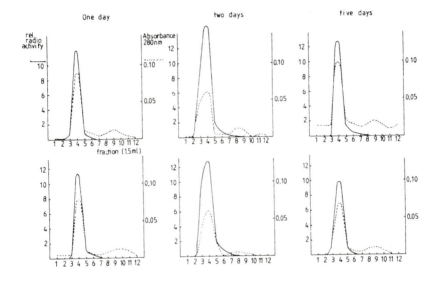

Figure 1. Sephadex G50 chromatography in In-111 labelled DTPA fibrinogen after 1,2 and 5 days' storage at 38°C. Upper part PBS as solvent, lower part 4.5% sucrose in PBS as solvent.

Figure 2 shows the relation between storage time and specific activity of the main protein fractions showing that there is no decrease in specific activity of the indium labelled DTPA fibrinogen.

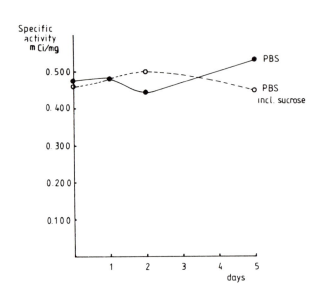

Figure 2. Specific activity of In-111-DTPA fibrinogen after storage at 38°C for five days.

Stability of monoclonal antibody (115 D8)-DTPA labelled with In-111 oxinate.

Monoclonal antibody DTPA In-111 elution profiles (chromatography on Sephadex G50 fine) are presented in Fig. 3.

The upper part shows the profiles if PBS is used as solvent. The middle part if 4.5% sucrose in PBS is used and the lower part if h.e.s. is used as potential stabilizing agent. It is clear that indium labelled 115 D8 is quite stable under the circumstances

312

studied and it hardly matters whether or not stabilizing agent is added as solvent, except for hydroxyethyl starch, which has destabilizing properties.

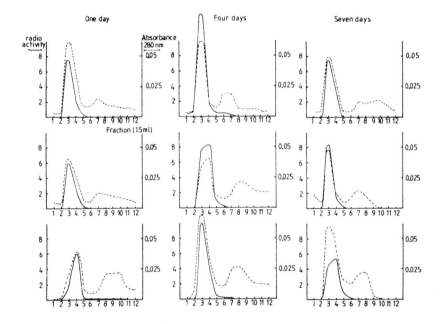

Figure 3. Sephadex G50 chromatograph of In-111 labelled 115D8 after 1,4 and 7 days' storage at 40°C.
Upper part PBS as solvent, middle 4.5 % sucrose (in PBS), lower part hydroxyethyl starch as solvent.

Figure 4 shows the relation between storage time and specific activity of the main protein fractions showing that there is some decrease in specific activity of the indium labelled DTPA m.c.a. after one day's storage but that at prolonged storage the m.c.a.

313

preparations are quite stable. Sucrose seems to be the appropriate stabilizing agent. H.e.s. is not suited as stabilizing agent.

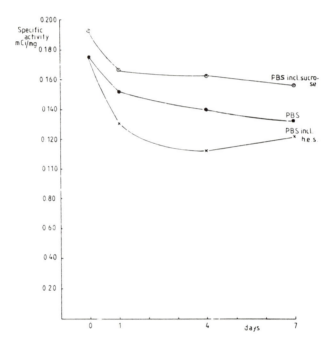

Figure 4. Specific activity of In-111 DTPA monoclonal antibody after storage at 40°C for 7 days.

Biological testing (elisa) of 115 D8, whether or not modified by

DTPA coupling and labelled with In-111, revealed that after 7 days' storage still significant biological activity was present. Quantitatively there was an obvious decrease, however this decrease was similar for antibody labelled and antibody unmodified indicating that DTPA coupling and labelling with In-111 did not contribute to the thermal (in)stability of the monoclonal antibody.

Stability of albumin-DTPA-In-111 in presence of Fe-59 ; possible exchange of In-111 by Fe-59?

In the circulation of a warm blooded animal, radiolabelled protein is surrounded by a tremendous amount of iron connected to proteins, mainly transferrins.

One of the prerequisites of stability of the radiolabelled proteins in the circulation is that iron in the circulation cannot exchange with indium and as such drives out the tracer from the protein molecule. We already know that the specific activity of the labelled protein does not significantly decrease after storage at $40^{\circ}C$, but this was not done in an excess of iron and the statistical variation of specific activity determinations does not completely rule out the possibility that a limited amount of iron could exchange indium for the protein molecule. To test this possibility we used Fe-59 as competitive ion in the stability testing. For technical reasons we did not use serum as a medium for incubation. We then run into trouble when separating the labelled protein from other serum proteins containing free tracer. We incubated the labelled protein, in fact human albumin, in an aqueous solution;where Fe-59 was present as citrate and incubated for 65 hours at $40^{\circ}C$. Radioactive indium and Fe-59 can separately be measured because of the good discrimination between the 1099

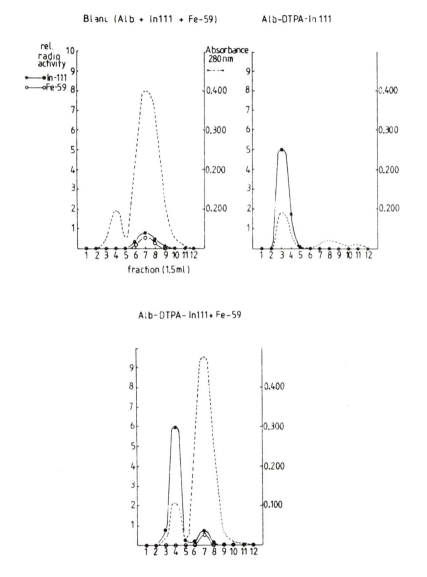

Figure 5. Elution profiles of gel chromatographic separations of In-111 labelled albumin samples after incubation with Fe-59 citrate for 65 hours at 40°C.

and 1292 KeV peaks of Fe-59 and the 245 and 171 KeV peaks of In-111, if measured on a Ge-Li scintillation detector.

Before incubation with Fe-59 citrate Indium-111 labelled DTPA albumin was incubated with cold Fe citrate for 20 minutes at 40°C to occupy empty DTPA sites.

Elution profiles (Sephadex G50 chromatograph) of albumin-In-111 + Fe-59, albumin DTPA-In-111 and albumin-DTPA-In-111 + Fe-59 are shown in Figure 5. The big peaks (dotted line), fractions 7 of the blank and Alb-DTPA-In-111 + Fe-59, are Fe citrate which separately from the albumin peaks (fraction 4) eluted from the column. Optically there is good attachment of In-111 to albumin (Alb-DTPA-In-111 and Alb-DTPA-In-111+Fe59) and there is no coupling of Fe-59 to albumin. So Fe-59 is not able to drive In-111 away from the DTPA coordination sites.

Quantitatively the results could be expressed as follows:

16 nCi Fe-59 or 0.3% of the Fe-59 radioactivity offered, coupled to albumin-DTPA-In-111. Including carrier Fe, this was 1.2×10^{13} atoms. These atoms were unable to push aside 1.3×10^{12} Indium-111 atoms (99 uCi In-111) already present on 0.5 mg protein.

So exchange did not take place with In-111.

2.6 nCi Fe-59 that is 0.05% of the Fe-59 radioactivity offered, coupled to the albumin blank. So a specific binding was neglectable. Specific activity of Alb-DTPA-In-111 after 65 hours at 40°C was 189 uCi/mg; of Alb-DTPA-In + Fe-59 after 65 hours 174 uCi/mg. This difference is within statistical limits due to the inaccuracy of the assay.

DISCUSSION

Stability testing of In-111 DTPA fibrinogen and In-111 DTPA monoclonal antibody indicates that DTPA is firmly connected to the protein and that the chelate bond between Indium and DTPA is not significantly impaired despite the loss of one carboxyl group in the formation of the amide bond with the amino group of lysine in the protein molecule. In case of labelled m.c.a. there is a drop of about 20 % specific activity after one day's storage at 40°C.

We ascribe this as loss of indium from the protein molecule which was aspecifically bound and was not immediately removed by gel chromatography. Storage of a biological active protein at 40°C for 7 days is quite a burden and we are not disappointed by losing some biological activity as measured by the elisa test. On the contrary we were happy to find still significant biological activity present in the m.c.a. preparation. As the decrease in biological activity was similar for unmodified antibody we concluded that DTPA modification with consecutively labelling with In-111 did not affect the stability of the monoclonal antibody.

In general there is no need to use a stabilizer in protein-DTPA preparations. Sucrose showed some stabilizing effect in case of m.c.a., but we doubt if addition of this compound is really necessary. H.e.s. has no stabilizing effect at all.

Fe-59 does not exchange with In-111 on albumin-DTPA labelled with In-111, however, the binding of Fe-59 to this protein is considerably higher than to the albumin blank without DTPA (16nCi versus 2.6 nCi). We think that this phenomenon can be explained by exchange of Fe-59 by cold Fe or cadmium (an impurity of In-111 preparations) which occupy the majority of the DTPA coordination sites on the protein molecule. This would result in a limited decrease of specific In-111 activity on the protein, an effect that we indeed observed, but technical limitations on specific activity measurement make this conclusion speculative.

Another possibility is that this difference is only a matter of different tailing by a not complete separation of the different peaks.

Concluding, we assume that indium coupling to DTPA modified proteins is sufficiently firm to allow tracer studies of those labelled proteins in warm blooded animals.

In fact the proof of this statement, with respect to In-111 labelled m.c.a. against human milk fat globule antigen used for breast tumour imaging in nude mice, is decribed elsewhere (Haisma et al 1984).

REFERENCES

- Benisek, W.F. and Richards, F.M. Attachment of metal-chelating Functional Groups to Hen Egg White Lysozyme. J. Biol. Chem. 243: 4267-4271 (1968).

- Eckelman, W.C., Karesh, S.M. and Reba, R.C.J. New compounds: fatty acid and long chain hydrocarbon derivatives containing a strong chelating agent. J. Pharm. Sci 64: 704-706 (1975).

- Goedemans, W.Th., Simplified cell labelling with Indium-111 acetylacetonate and Indium-111 oxinate. Brit. J. Rad. 54:636-637 (1981).

- Goedemans W. Th., Method of preparing radionuclide-labelled proteins in particular antibodies or antibody fragments. Patent application to be published.

- Gokce, A., Nakamura, R.M., Tubis, M. and Wolf, W. Synthesis of Indium-labelled Antibody-chelate Conjugates for Radioassays Int. J. Nucl. Med. Biol.9:85-95 (1982).

- Haisma, H., Goedemans, W.Th. and Hilkens, J. Improved tumour imaging using subtraction of Indium labelled specific and gallium labelled non-specific antibody. International Symposium on Immunoscintigraphy, Saariselka, Lapland, August 10-12th, (1984).

- Hilkens, J., Hilgers, J. Hageman, Ph., Buijs, F., van Doornewaard, G., Schol, D. and Atsma D. Monoclonal antibodies against milkfat globule membrane antigens; Their usefulness in human carcinoma pathology Protides of the Biological Fluids Brussels-Belgium May 2 - May 5, 1983.

- Hnatowich, D.J., Layne, W.W. and Childs, R.L. The Preparation and Labelling of DTPA-coupled Albumin. Int. J. Appl. Radiat. Isot. 33: 327-332 (1982).

- Hnatowich, D.J., Layne, W.W., Childs, R.L., Lanteigne, D., Davis, M.A., Griffin, T.W. and Doherty P.W. radioactive Labelling of Antibody: A simple and efficient Method. Science 220: 613-615 (1983).

- Janoki, A.GY., Harwig, J.F. and Wolf W. Studies on high specific activity labelling of proteins using bifunctional chelates: Ga-67-DF-HSA. Nuclear Medicine and Biology. Proc. Third. World Congress Paris 689-692 (1982).

- Janoki, GY.A., Harwig, J.F. Chanachai, W., and Wolf W. (^{67}Ga) Desferrioxamine-HSA: Synthesis of Chelon Protein Conjugates using Carbodiimide as a Coupling Agent. Int. J. Appl. Radiat. Isot. 34: 871-877 (1983).

- Khaw, B.A., Fallon, J.T., Strauss, H.W. and Haber, E.. Myocardial Infarct Imaging of Antibodies to Canine Cardiac Myosin with Indium-111-Diethylene triamine Penta acetic Acid. Science 209: 295:297 (1980).

- Krejcarek and Tucker K., Covalent attachment of chelating groups to macromolecules. Biochem. Biophys, Res. Commun. 77:581-585 (1977).

- Layne W.W., Hnatowich, D.M., Doherty, P.W., Childs, R.L., Lanteigne, D., and Ansell, J. Evaluation of the Viability of In-111-Labelled DTPA Coupled to Fibrinogen. J. Nucl. Med., 23: 627-630 (1982).

- Ohmomo, Y., Yohoyama, A., Suzuki, J., Tanaka, H., Yamamoto, K., Horiuchi K., Ishii, Y. and Torizuka, K., Eur. J. Nucl. Med. 7: 458-461 (1982).

- Sundberg, M.W., Meares, C.F., Goodwin, D.A. and Diamanti, C.I. Selective binding of metal ions to macromolecules using bifunctional analogs of EDTA. J. Med. Chem. 17: 1304-1307 (1974).

- Wolf W., Gokce, A., Tubis, M. and O'Brien, J. U.S. Patent 4, 320, 109 March 16, 1982.

- Yokoyama, A., Aramo, Y., Hosotani, T., Yamada, A., Horiuchi, K., Yamanoto, K., Torizuka, K., Ueda, M. and Hazue M. Introducing new 99m-Tc-bifunctional Radiopharmaceutical containing dithiosemicarbazone chelate group. Nuclear Medicine and Biology Proc. Third World Congress Paris 1097-1100 (1982).

- Yokoyama, A., Ohmomo, Y., Horiuchi, K., Saji, H., Tanaka, H., Yamamoto, K., Ishii, Y. and Torizuka, K., Desferoxamine, A promising Bifunctional Chelating Agent for Labelling Proteins with Gallium: Ga-67 DF-HSA. Consise Communication J. Nucl. Med. 23: 909-914 (1982).

Heterogeneity of Human Milk Fat Globulin Antigens, revealed by Monoclonal Antibodies

Krohn K.[1], Ashorn P.[1], Helle M.[2] and Ashorn R.[1]

(1) Institute of Biomedical Sciences, University of Tampere, Finland.

(2) Mikkeli Central Hospital, Mikkeli, Finland.

Correspondence: Dr. Krohn K., M.D., Institute of Biomedical Sciences, University of Tampere, P.O. Box 607, 33101 Tamper 10, Finland.

INTRODUCTION

Human milk fat globules (HMFS) are known to contain antigenic structures that are expressed, in addition to normal or lactating breast, in a variety of malignancies (3, 1, 7, 10). Because of this, antibodies against HMFG have been used in the histological or cytological diagnosis of cancer (7, 19, 6). More recently they have also been used in setting prognosis after mastectomy (21), and in attempted therapy in patients with advanced carcinomas (8).

Milk fat globules are generally believed to carry membrane antigens similar to the membranes of the lactating cells. Polyclonal antisera may therefore react with several different molecules on the membrane. Monoclonal antibodies, recognizing only one epitope, should be expected to have a more strict specificity. Hypothetically, some monoclonal antibodies could recognize epithelial cells, the other cells with proliferative or metabolic activity. Against the odds, this has not been the case, suggesting that similar epitopes are present in several carrier molecules.

We have previously described the production of a series of monoclonal antibodies against HMFG, with some of the antibodies reacting with 100%, one antibody (III D 5) only with 70% of mammary or ovarian carcinomas. The latter 70% consisted mainly of estrogen receptor positive cases. Here we describe characterization of antigenic determinants recognized by different monoclonal antibodies against HMFG using western blotting.

MATERIALS AND METHODS

Preparation of HMFG membrane antigens.

Fresh human milk was divided into cream and skim milk by centrifugation for 30 min. at 2000 rpm. The extraction of HMFG antigens was carried out as described elsewhere (3). The lyophilized HMFG was stored in freeze-dried form at $+4^{\circ}C$, skim milk and its fractions at $-20^{\circ}C$.

Preparation of antibodies

Production of monoclonal antibodies against HMFG has been described previously (12), using BALB/c mice and SP-2 myeloma cells. Primary screening was with ELISA (see below), and supernatants from positive clones were further tested with IFL, using mammary or ovarian carcinoma cells as target cells. These were obtained from peritoneal or pleural effusions from advanced cancer patients; antibodies reacting with cancer cells but not with lymphocytes, monocytes or mesothelial cells present in the effusions were used in further studies. In this paper we described

324

the use of four such monoclonal antibodies, III H 2, III E 8, III C 12 and III D 5.

Fractionation of skim milk

30 ml of skim milk was concentrated by ultrafiltration and fractionated on a 2.5 x 100 cm Sephacryl S-300 column (Pharmacia Fine Chemicals, Uppsala, Sweden). 5 ml fractions were eluted with 0.1 M Tris-EDTA buffer, pH 8.0 and the protein concentration was measured by absorbance at 280 nm. HMFG-antigen activity was assayed by ELISA whereafter the fractions were combined into pools I, II and III, and concentrated by ultrafiltration.

Immunohistochemistry

Surgical and gynecological specimens were fixed in 10% neutral formalin, embedded in paraffin and sections were stained with heamatoxylin-eosin and with the monoclonal antibodies. Endogenous peroxidase was blocked by 3% methanol. Monoclonal antibodies (ascites fluid) were diluted 1:100 and secondary antibody, peroxidase conjugated rabbit anti-mouse immunoglobulin (Dakopats, Copenhagen, Denmark) in 1:40. Ethylene aminocarbazol was used as a substrate and the sections were counter-stained with haemalum.

Steroid receptor assays

Immediately after removal of the tumour block, a representative piece of cancer tissue (usually up to 2 g, if available) was removed and frozen in liquid nitrogen. Estrogen and progesterone receptor content of the tumour was then assessed by sytosol-biochemical method (4). A limit of a positive receptor status was > 5 fmol/mg of protein.

325

ELISA

Enzyme linked immmunosorbent assay was performed as described by Engwall (5). 100 ul of HMFG (10 ug/ml), skim milk (10 ug/ml) or undiluted fractions from Sephacryl S-300 were pipetted on ELISA plates (Dynatech Ag, 6300 Zug, Switzerland) and incubated overnight at $+4^{o}$C. Antibody incubations (60 min. at $+37^{o}$C, ascites diluted 10^{-3} in PBS-1% BSA) were followed by peroxidase-conjugated rabbit anti-mouse immunoglobulins (Miles Laboratories, Rehovot, Israel, dilution 1:400) and 1,2-phenylendiamindihydrochloride-substrate (Fluka Ag, Buchs Sg, Switzerland). The washings were with phosphate-buffered saline (pH 7.4), containing 0.05% Tween 20 (PBS-Tween). An automatic ELISA reader (Labsystems, Helskinki, Finland) was used in the recording.

SDS-PAGE and immunoblotting

For polyacrylamide gel electrophoresis the protocol of Laemmli (14) was used. Briefly, 20 ul of sample was diluted 1:5 in sample buffer and kept in boiling water for 5 min. Pretreated samples were then run in the SDS-acrylamide gel. The proteins were electrically transferred onto nitrocellulose sheet (Schleicher & Schull GmbH, Dassel, West-Germany) and stained with monoclonal antibodies (20), normally diluted 1:100 in Tris-buffer saline (TBS) containing 0.2% Triton X-100 (Sigma), pH 7.4. Staining with III D 5 antibody was done with dilution of 1:1000 in TBS without Triton X-100. Binding of antisera was detected by peroxidase-conjugated rabbit anti-mouse IgG (Miles Laboratories) dilution 1:400, followed by a 5 min. incubation with 4-chloronaphthole solution (Merck). The washings were 4 x 5 min. with TBS. The antigens on nitrocellulose paper were also stained with biotinylated Peanut agglutinine (Vector Laboratories, Inc., Burlingame, Ca., USA, dilution 1:120, incubation 60 min. at $+37^{\circ}C$), the binding of which was detected by incubation for 15 min. with peroxidase-conjugated avidin (Vector Laboratoires, dilution 1:2000), followed by the substrate. When the proteins were not transferred onto nitrocellulose paper, gels were stained either with Amido black (Merck) or periodic-acid-Schiff (PAS) as described by Fairbanks (9).

RESULTS

The reactivity of the monoclonal antibodies against skim milk and HMFG was first tested in ELISA. As can be seen in table 1, three of them (antibodies III C 12, III E 8 and III H 2) reacted more strongly against HMFG, one (III D 5) with skim milk.

Table 1. Reactivities of anti-HMFG monoclonal antibodies with skim milk and HMFG in ELISA.

Antibody	Antigen	
	Skim milk	HMGF
III C 12	0,108*	0.561
III D 5	0.790	0.673
III E 8	0.116	0.705
III H 2	0.125	0.664

* Optical density at 495 nm.

Immunohistochemistry

All four antibodies stained the luminal plasma membrane of normal, lactating or mastophathic breast epithelium (Figure 1). With mammary carcinomas, quantitative and qualitative differences were seen. Antibodies III H 2, III E 8 and III C 12 reacted with all primary carcinomas tested (Table 2). Staining was always membranous, and in contrast to benign cells, whole circumference of malignant cells were usually stained (Figure 2). Antibody III D 5 stained only c. 70 % of the primary mammary tumours; with this antibody, staining was always cytoplasmic, and coarsely granular (Figures 3 and 4).

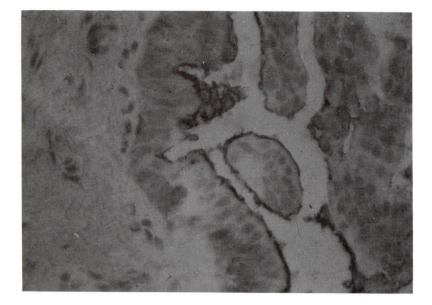

Figure 1 Reactivity of antibody III H 2 with normal breast

ductal epithelium.

Table 2. Immunohistochemical reactivity of different anti-HMFG antibodies in primary and metastatic mammary carcinomas.

Diagnosis	Antibody	Reactivity	
		Positive	Negative
Primary carcinoma	III D 5	34[a]	17
	III H 2	51	0
	III E 8	51	0
	III C 12	51	0
Metastases	III D 5	9	6
	III E 8	6	2

a) Number of cases

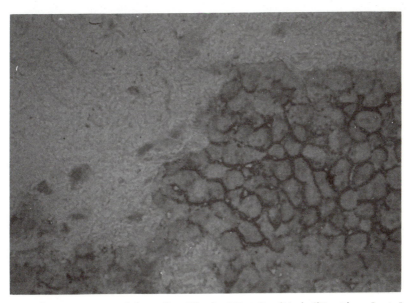

Figure 2. Reactivity of antibody III H 2 with infiltrating ductal

329

mammary carcinoma.

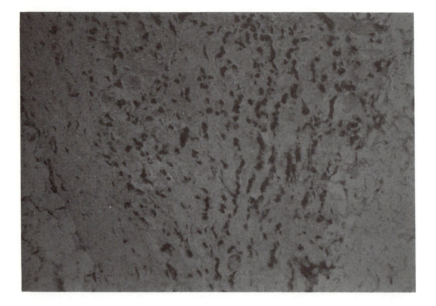

Figure 3. Reactivity of antibody III D 5 with infiltrating ductal mammary carconoma.

Metastatic lesions generally followed the staining characteristcs of the primary tumour (Figure 5 and Table 2). In some cases, however, metastatic cells were negative, even when most cells in the primary tumour were positive.

Correlation of immunohistochemistry and estrogen receptor status

The reaction of III D 5 antibody with mammary carcinomas were correlated with the estrogen (ER) and progesteron (PR) receptor status of the tumour. No correlation was seen with PR status. In contrast, staining with III D 5 correlated highly significantly with the ER status (Table 3). The borderline cases in the table showed only weak staining or less than 5% of tumour cells were positive.

Fractionation of skim milk

Skim milk was fractionated on Sephacryl S-300 and the reactivity of each fraction was tested with ELISA. Figure 6 shows the results using III D 5 antibody. The other antibodies gave a similar binding curve. The fractions were pooled as shown in figure and used in immunoblotting analysis.

Table 3. Correlation of anti-HMFG III D 5 reactivity to estrogen receptor status in primary mammary carcinoma.

Estrogen receptor

	Positive	Negative
III D 5 positive	25	4
III D 5 negative	4	12
III D 5 borderline	1	5

$p < 0.0001$, x^2

Western blotting

HMFG failed to enter the gel probably because of the high molecular weight of the antigens. In skim milk, however, several molecules of different sizes readily entered the gel. As shown in

331

figure 7, all the monoclonal antibodies visualized several antigens in skim milk, the majority of which were detectable by all the antibodies but one in the region of 42 to 57 kDa only with the antibody III D 5.

Western blotting analysis of skim milk pools I, II and III is shown in figure 8. The antigens reacting with III D 5 were located in the first peak containing the largest molecules, whereas those reacting with the others (III H 2, III E 8 and III C 12) mainly in pool II. Pool III, consisting of the smallest molecules, showed no reactivity against any of the antibodies. Staining with Amido black and Coomassie blue for protein and periodic-acid-Schiff and Peanut agglutinine for polysaccharides were used to further characterize the antigenic structures in skim milk. As shown in figure 9, all the antigens except the one in the region of 42 to 57 kDa can be stained with a protein dye. Four molecules can be stained with periodic-acid-Schiff and those plus still give more bound Peanut agglutinine (PNA).

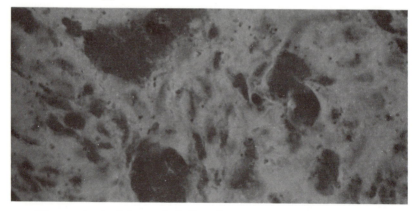

Figure 4. Staining of infiltraing ductal mammary carcinoma with antibody III D 5 showing coarsely granular intracytoplasmic reactivity.

332

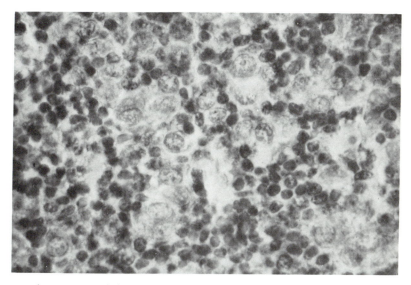

Figure 5 Staining of metastatic mammary carcinoma cels in lymph node with antibody III D 5.

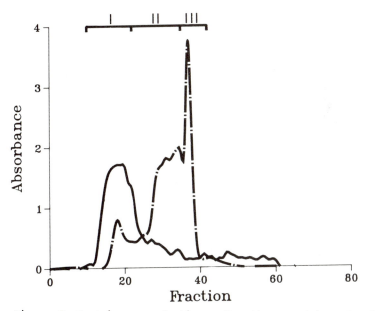

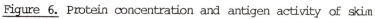

Figure 6. Protein concentration and antigen activity of skim

milk fractions from Sephacryl S-300. The dotted line indicates absorbance at 280 nm and the solid one reactivity against anti-HMFG antibody in ELISA. Pooling of the fractions is marked above.

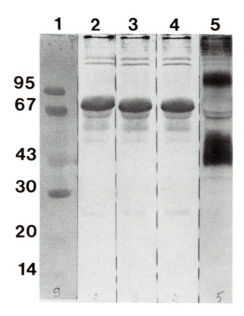

Figure 7. Immunoblotting of skim milk. Samples were run in SDS-PAGE, transferred onto nitrocellulose sheet and stained with monoclonal antisera III H 2 (land 2) III E 8 (Lane 3), III C 12 Lane 4) III D 5 (Lane 5). Positions of molecular marker proteins (MW/kDa) are shown in lane 1.

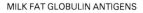

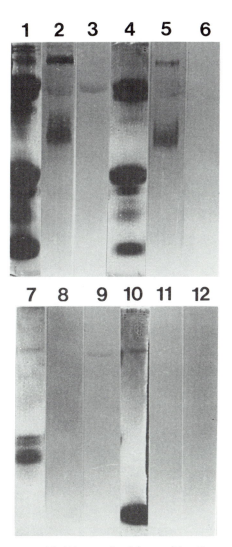

Figure 8. Immunoblotting of skim milk (lanes 1–3)and its fractions from Sepharcryl S-3000: pool I (lanes 4–6), pool II (lanes 7–9) and pool III (lanes 10–12). Staining was with Amido black (lanes 1,4,7 and 10) monoclonal antibody III D 5 (lanes 2,5,8,11) and monoclonal antibody III H 2 (lanes 3,6,9,12)

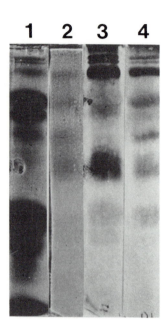

Figure 9. Staining of skim milk components with 1) Amido black, 2) periodic-acid-Schiff, 3) monoclonal antibody III D 5 and 4) Peanut agglutinine.

DISCUSSION

In the present work we wanted to characterize the antigenic epitopes detected by monoclonal antibodies against HMFG. Of special interest was antibody III D 5, which detects antigenic molecules in mammary carcinomas, the expression of which seems to correlate with estrogen receptor status of the tumour. The other three antibodies, III H 2, III E 8 and III C 12, have similar immunohistochemical reactivity as anti-HMFG monoclonal antibodies described by others (18) with wide use in immunoscintigraphy (6)(7) and possibly also as curative agents (8) and are therefore also of interest.

Although the primary interest with tumour associated monoclonal antibodies is in the antigenic epitopes present in the malignant cells, products of the normal cells, in this case milk, is a convenient material in characterization of the nature of the antibodies. Our antibodies were originally generated against HMFG. However, all the antibodies also reacted with skim milk and in ELISA, antibody III D 5 even more strongly than with the immunizing agent. This can be due to contamination of the antigen used in the immunization. Another explanation is that skim milk contains smaller fat globules, skim milk globules, carrying similar antigenic structure to milk fat globules. These globules might be produced independently from HMFG secretion or they could be degradation products from larger fat globules as suggested by Ormerod (16).

When fractionating with a Sephacryl S-300 column, the antigenic activity was eluted in the void volume. This indicates a molecular weight of > 1500 kDa supporting the theory that the epitopes detected by the antibodies are located on larger particles in skim milk, skim milk globules. Our preliminary results show that if ion-exchange chromatography is used, the epitopes responsible for the antigen antibody reaction are separated into several pools. This suggest that antigenic subunits carry identical determinants but also others that differ from each other in electrical charges, possible due to variable amounts of glycosylation of phosphorylation.

The model of a large molecule consisting of several smaller antigenic subunits fits well with the immunoblotting results. We have one antigen detectable with antibody III D 5 and others detectable by all the antibodies. As antibody III D 5 also shows a different histochemistry and a relation to the estrogen receptor, we can draw a conclusion that at least two different epitopes have to be present in the same molecule and, on the other hand, similar epitopes are found in different molecules. This is well in keeping with the idea that skim milk contains small fat droplets enveloped in similar membrame structures to the larger milk fat globules. The density of these skim milk globules may be just between that of cream and skim milk making it difficult to toally separate them from either fractions in simple centrifugations.

What comes to the molecule exclusively stained with antibody III D 5, a low polypeptide concentration and presence of galactosamine and an acetylgalactosamine residues were shown, indicated by positive staining with PAS and PNA. It is especially interesting that this molecule binds PNA, as this feature has been shown to correlate positively with the estrogen receptor status in breast cancers (2). In addition PNA staining is suggested to be a marker for breast epithelial cell differentiation (15) and a possible link between neoplastic transformation and the development of tumour immunity (11). A more detailed study about lectin binding affinities of HMFG antigens is being carried out and will be published later by us.

All HMFG-antibody preparations, described so far, have reacted with normal tissue in addition to malignant cells. None of these antibodies can therefore be considered carcinoma specific. The observed heterogeneity of the antigenic structures, recognized by different monoclonal and polyclonal antibodies, makes it however possible, that some of the many HMFG-associated antigenic epitopes might be more strongly expressed in the malignant cells. A panel of several monoclonal antibodies, possible generated against purified antigenic structures, may therefore prove to be useful tool in immunohistochemical tumour diagnosis and in immunoscintigraphy as well.

REFERENCES

1. Arklie J., Taylor-Papadimitriou J., Bodmer W., Egan M. and Millis R. (1981): Differentiation antigens expressed by epithelial cells in the lactating breast are also detectable in breast cancers. Int. J. Cancer 28, 23–29.

2. Bocker W., Klaubert A., Bahnsen J., Schweikhart G., Pollow K., Mitze M., Kreinberg R., Beck T. and Stegner H.E. (1984): Peanut lectin histochemistry of 120 mammary carcinomas and its relation to tumour type, grading, staging, and receptor status. Virchows Arch. (Pathol. Anat.) 403, 149–161.

3. Ceriani R., Thompson K., Peterson J. and Abraham S. (1977): Surface differentiation antigens of human mammary epithelial cells carried on the human milk fat globule. Proc. Natl. Acad. Sci. 74, 582–586.

4. Edwards D.P., Chamness G.C. and McGuire W.L. (1979): Estrogen and progesterone proteins in breast cancer. Biochim. Biophys. Acta 560, 457–486.

5. Engwall E. and Perlman P. (1971): Enzymelinked immunosorbent assay (ELISA). Quantative assay of immunoglobulin G. Immunohistochemistry 8, 871–874.

6. Epenetos A., Canti G., Taylor-Papadimitriou J., Curling M. and Bodmer W. (1982a): Use of two epithelium-spesific monoclonal antibodies for diagnosis of malignancy in serous effusions. Lancet 11 (8306), 1004–1006.

7. Epenetos A., Mather S., Granowska M., Nimmon C., Hawkins L., Britton K., Shepherd J., Taylor-Papadinitriou J., Durbin H. and

Malpas J. (1982b): Targetting of iodine-123-labelled tumour-associated monoclonal antibodies to ovarian, breast and gastrointestinal tumours. Lancet 11 (8306), 1001–1004.

8. Epenetos A., Halnan K., Hooker G., Highes J., Krausz T., Lambert J., Lavender J., MacGregor W., McKenzie C., Munro A., Myers M., Orr J., Pearse E., Snook D. and Webb B. (1984): Antibody-guided irradiation of malignant lesions: three cases illustrating a new method of treatment. Lancet 6 (8392), 1441–1443.

9. Fairbaks G., Steck T. and Wallach D. (1971): Electrophoretic analysis of the major polypeptides of the human erythrocyte membrane. Biochemistry 10, 2606–2617.

10. Hilkens J., Buijs F., Hilgers J., Hageman Ph., Calafat J., Sonnenberg A. and Valk van der M. (1984): Monoclonal antibodies against human milk-fat globule membranes detecting differentiation antigen of the mammary gland and its tumours. Int. J. Cancer 34, 197–206.

11. Howard D. and Batsakis J. (1980): Cytostructural localization of a tumour-associated antigen. Science 210, 201–203.

12. Krohn K., Ashorn R. and Helle M. (1984a): Generation of monoclonal antibodies to milk fat globulin membrane antigens, with sepcial reference to a precipitable secretory product of breast and ovarial carcinomas. Submitted for publication.

13. Krohn K., Ashorn R. and Helle M. (1984b): Detection with a monoclonal antibody an estrogen receptor associated antigen in mammary and ovarial carcinomas. Protides of the Biological Fluids, in press.

14. Laemmli U. (1970): Cleavage of structural proteins during the assembly of the head of bacteriophage T4. Nature 227, 680–685.

340

15. Newman R., Klein P. and Rudland P. (1979): Binding of peanut lectin to breast epithelium, human carcinomas and a cultured rat mammary stem cell: use of lectin as a marker of mammary differentiation. JNCI 63, 1339–1346.

16. Ormerod M., Steele K., Westwood J. and Mazzini M. (1983): Epithelial membrane antigen: Partial purification, assay and properties. Br. J. Cancer 48, 533–541.

17. Sloane J. and Ormerod G. (1981): Distribution of epithelial membrane antigen in normal and neoplastic tissues and its value in diagnostic tumour pathology. Cancer 47, 1786–1795.

18. Taylor-Papdimitriou J., Peterson J., Arklie J., Burchell J. and Ceriani R. (1981): Monoclonal antibodies to epithelium-specific component of the human milk fat globule membrane: production and reaction with cells in culture. Int. J. Cancer 28, 17–21.

19. To A., Coleman D., Dearnaley D., Ormerod M., Steele K. and Neville A (1981): Use of antisera to epithelial membrane antigen for the cytodiagnosis of malignancy in serous effusions. J. Clin. Pathol. 34, 1326–1332.

20. Towbin H., Stahelin T. and Gordon J., (1979): Electrophoretic transfer of proteins from polyacrylamide gels to nitrocellulose sheets: Procedure and some applications. Proc. Natl. Acad. Sci. 76.4350–4354.

21. Wilkinson M., Howell A., Taylor-Papdimitriou J., Swindell R. and Sellwood R. (1984): The prognostic significance of two epithelial membrane antigens expressed by human mammary carcinomas. Int. J. Cancer 33, 299–304.

Emission Computerized Tomography (ECT) and I-123 Labelled fragments of Monoclonal Anti-cea Antibodies for the detection of Human Colorectal Carcinomas

Delaloye B., Bischof-Delaloye A., Buchegger F., Grob J.P. von
Fliedner V., Carrel S. and Mach J.P.

Division of Nuclear Medicine, Chuv, 1011 Lausanne,
Switzerland and Ludwig Institute for Cancer Research, 1066
Epalinges, Switzerland.

INTRODUCTION

The old dream of many tumour immunlogists, to find antibodies capable of detecting in vivo the hidden cancer cells has been revitalized by the development of monoclonal antibody (Mab) technology (1). This technique allowed the production in unlimited amounts of antibodies of perfect homgeneity and specificity directed against various tumour markers. In this brief review, we shall critically consider the use of radiolabelled antibodies as tracer for tumour detection, starting from our early experimental results with ^{131}I labelled polyclonal antibodies against carcinoembryonic antigen (CEA) up to the most recent clinical results obtained with ^{123}I labelled fragments of anti-CEA Mab. Special emphasis will be given to the difficulties encountered in the detection of liver metastases when using intact anti-CEA antibodies and to the improvement obtained by using ^{123}I labelled Mab fragments and emission computerized tomography (ECT) for their three dimensional localization.

EXPERIMENTAL RESULTS WITH POLYCLONAL ANTIBODIES

Research on tumour localization of radiolabelled antibodies was initiated almost 30 years ago by Pressman (2) and Bale (3), who showed that labelled antibodies against Wagner osteosarcoma or Walker carcinoma cells were concentrated in vivo by these tumours.

In 1974, we introduced into this field the model of nude mice bearing grafts of human colon carcinoma and these use of affinity purified antibodies against carcinoembryonic antigen (CEA)(4). We showed that purified ^{131}I-labelled goat anti-CEA antibodies could reach up to a 9 times higher concentration in the tumour than in the liver, while the concentration of control normal IgG in the tumour was never higher than 2.3 times that in the liver. We observed, however, great variations in the degree of specific tumour localization by the same preparation of labelled antibodies, when colon carcinoma grafts derived from different patients were tested. This is probably due to the fact that human tumours keep their initial histologic properties and degree of differentiation after transplantation into nude mice and these two factors appear to affect the ease with which circulating antibodies gain access to the CEA present in tumours. The detection of ^{131}I-labelled antibodies in tumours by external scanning also gave variable results. With colon carcinoma grafts from certain donors we obtained scans with good tumour localization, such as the one shown in fig. 1A whereas with colon carcinoma grafts from other donors the antibody uptake was not sufficient to give satisfactory scanning images. In this context, we think that results in the nude mouse model are a good reflection of the clinical reality observed in patients.

Independently, Goldenberg et al (5) showed specific tumour localization and detection by external scanning with ^{131}I-labelled IgG fractions of anti-CEA serum, using two human carcinomas which had been serially transplanted into hamsters for several years.

CLINICAL RESULTS WITH POLYCLONAL ANTI-CEA ANTIBODIES

The first detection of carcinoma in patients obtained by external scanning following injection of purified ^{131}I-labelled anti-CEA antibodies was reported by Goldenberg et al (6,7). They claimed that almost all the CEA producing tumours could be detected by this method and that there was no false positive results. However, our experience, using highly purified goat anti-CEA antibodies and the same blood pool subtraction technique as Goldenberg was that only 42% of CEA producing tumours (22 out of 53 tested) could be detected by this method (8-9). Furthermore, we found that in several patients the labelled anti-CEA antibodies localized non-specifically in the reticuloendothelium particularly in the liver. Despite the use of the subtraction technique, this non-specific uptake was difficult to differentiate from the specific uptake in liver metastases. The discrepancy of results between the group of Goldenberg and our own is unlikely to be due to a difference in the quality of the anti-CEA antibodies used, since we showed by direct measurement of the readioactivity in tumours resected after injection that our antibodies were capable of excellent tumour localization (8). Furthermore, in a few patients scheduled for tumour resection, we injected simultaneously 1 mg of goat anti-CEA antibodies labelled

345

with 1 m Ci of ^{131}I and 1 mg of control normal goat IgG labelled with 0.2 m Ci of ^{125}I. By this paired labelled method adapted to the patient situation, we could demonstrate that the antibody uptake was 4 times higher than that of control normal IgG (8).

These results were very encouraging in terms of specificity of tumour localization. However, the direct measurement of radioactivity in tumours also showed that only 0.05–0.2& of the injected radioactivity (0.5–2 uCi out of 1000 uCi) were recovered in the resected tumours 3–8 days after injection (8). This information is importanty if one is consering the use of ^{131}I labelled antibody for therapy (10).

MONOCLONAL ANTI-CEA ANTIBODIES USED IN IMMUNOSCINTIGRAPHY

The obvious advantage of monoclonal antibodies (Mab) are their homogeneity and their specificity for the immunizing antigen. Another advantage of Mab is that they each react with a single antigenic determinant and thus should not be able to form large immune complexes with the antigen (provided that the antigenic determinant is not repetitive).

The first Mab used for immunoscintigraphy in patients was Mab 23 anti-CEA (11). Already in 1981, the well characterized Mab 23 (12) was injected intravenously to 26 patients with large bowel carcinomas and 2 patients with pancreatic carcinomas. Each patient received 0.3 mg of purfied Mab labelled with 1–1.5 m Ci of ^{131}I. The patient's premedication included lugol 5 % iodine solution, promethazine and prednisolone, as previously described (8,9). The patients had no personal history of allergy. They were also tested with an intracutaneous injection of normal mouse IgG and found to have no hypersensitivity against this protein. None of the patients showed any sign of discomfort during or after the injection of labelled mouse antibodies. The patients were studied by static external photoscanning 24, 36, 48 and 72 h after injection. In 14 of the 28 patients (50 %) a hot area corresponding to the tumour was detected 36-48 h after injection. In 6 patients the scans were doubtful and the remaining 8 patients they were entirely negative (11).

The results were slightly better than those obtained with polyclonal anti-CEA antibodies (8,9). Namely there was less background radioactivity in the liver, but the method could not yet be considered as clinically useful in comparison with the other modern methods of tumour diagnosis.

DETECTION OF COLORECTAL CARCINOMA BY TOMOSCINTIGRAPHY

A logical approach to improve tumour detection by immunoscintigraphy is the use of tomoscintigraphy. As we have seen, planar on imaging is limited in part of the presence of radiolabelled antibodies or free [131] released from them, in the circulation, the reticuloendothelial system, the stomach, intestine and urinary bladder. Increased radioactivity in these compartments may give false positive results. Tumour sites may be masked by sites of non-specific uptakes. These problems cannot be entirely resolved by the presently available subtraction methods using ^{99m}Tc labelled HSA and ^{99m}Tc pertechnetate. Axial transverse tomoscintigraphy is a method initially developed by Kuhl and Edwards already in 1963 (13) with the potential to resolve some of these problems. This method, also called single photon emission computerized tomography (SPECT) or (ECT) is based on the reconstruction of transverse, coronal or sagittal sections from

347

series of scintigraphic views taken at different angles around the patient. Similar mathematical techniques are used in positron or X-ray tomography. In collaboration with Ch. Berche and J.D. Lumbroso from the Institut Gustave Roussy in Ville juif, we have shown that tomoscintigraphy can improve the sensivity and specificity of tumour detection by radiolabelled anti-CEA Mabs (11,14). With this methods 15 out of 16 carcinoma tumour sites studied (including 10 colorectal carcinomas, 1 stomach, 1 pancreas and 4 medullary thyroid carcinomas) were detectable. These results were encouraging in term of sensitivity. However, it should be noted that numerous non-specific radioactive hot areas, sometimes as intense as the tumours, were observed. Thus, the problem of non-specific accumulation of antibodies remained, but the three dimensional localization of radioactive spots by tomoscintigraphy helped to discriminate specific tumour uptakes from the non-specific ones. Another problem was that relatively thick sections of 2.5 cm were required because the number of events (counts) were too low for statistical analysis of thinner sections. Furthermore the spatial resolution was low due the high energy of ^{131}I (14).

RESULTS

MAB FRAGMENTS TESTED IN EXPERIMENTAL ANIMALS

In order to further improve this method, we produced a series of 26 new hybridomas secreting anti-CEA antibodies and selected them first, in vitro, by criteria of high affinity for CEA (15) and low crossreactivity with glycoproteins present on the surface of granulocytes, termed NCA-55 and NCA-95 (16). Furthermore, $F(ab')_2$ and Fab fragments were prepared from three selected Mab

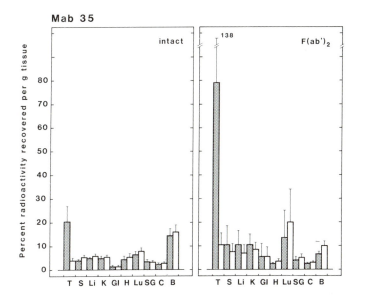

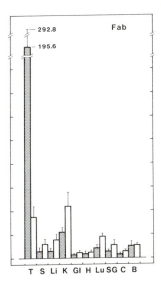

Figure 1: Distribution of Mab 35 or its fragments (shaded bars) and control IgG or fragments (open bars) injected simultaneously into nude mice bearing grafts of a human carcinoma. The vertical lines represent the standard deviation calculated from groups of four to seven animals per Mab or fragment . T,tumour; S, Spleen; Li, liver; k, kidneys; GI,gastrointestinal tract; H, heart; Lu, lungs; SG, salivary glands; C, carcass and head; B, blood. (reproduced with the permission of the J. Exp. Med.) (17).

and tested for their capacity to localize, in vivo, in human colon carcinoma heterotransplanted in nude mice (17). Groups of 4-7 mice were injected simultaneously with ^{131}I labelled Mab or fragments and with normal IgG or their corresponding fragment labelled with ^{125}I. The mice were dissected 2-5 days later. The results of antibody and normal IgGconcentration per g of tumour and normal organ obtained with Mab 35 and expressed in percentage of the total radioactivity recovered for each isotope are shown in Figure 1.

It is evident that the ratios of tumour to normal organ antibody concentration is increasing dramatically with the use of fragments. The ratios of tumour to normal organ antibody concentration (average from all normal organ) were 7 for intact Mab, 25 for F(ab')$_2$ and 85 for Fab. The specificity indices calculated by dividing the tumour to normal organs ratios obtained for antibody by the corresponding ratio obtained for control IgG were 3.4 for intact Mab, 8.2 for F(ab')$_2$ and 19 for Fab (17).

The scanning results obtained with these experimental animals were in agreement with those obtained by direct measurement of radioactivity. With intact Mab tumour grafts of 0.5-1 g gave contrasted positive scans only 3 days after injection, whereas fragments of Mab allowed the detection of smaller tumours at an earlier time. The best results were obtained with Fab fragments of Mab 35 which allowed the clear detection of a tumour graft of 0.1 g 48 h after injection (17). Figure 1 compares the scans obtained with intact polyclonal anti-CEA antibodies in 1974 (4) (panel A) with those obtained recently with FAb fragments of Mab 35 (17) (panel B).

DETECTION OF CARCINOMA USING $\underline{^{131}}$I LABELLED MAB

FRAGMENTS AND ECT

Based on the above experimental results, a series of 23 patients with colorectal carcinoma were tested after injection of F(ab')2 and Fab fragments of Mab 35 labelled with ^{123}I. This isotope, which has a very favorable energy of 159 Kev and a relatively short physical half life of 13.2 hours, proved to be excellent for tomoscintigraphy. ^{123}I was prepared from the ^{127}I(p,5n) ^{123}Xe reaction and provided by the Schweizerisches Institut fur Reaktorforschung at Wurenlingen, Switzerland. Using a Siemens dual head rotating camera, tomographic studies of the pelvis and upper abdomen were performed in all patients at 6 h and 24 h after injection and in the majority of patients at 48 h. Other parts of the body such as thorax and bones were studied only when there was a clinical suspicion of tumour in these areas or when an abnormal radioactive uptake was detected on the whole body scan systematically performed before the tomographic studies. No subtraction techniques were used, but additional scintigraphic studies of the liver with ^{99m}Tc sulfur colloid were regularly performed after the last ^{123}I analysis of the upper abdomen with the patient remaining in the same position. Sulfur colloid scintigraphy allowed identification of anatomical landmarks and in some cases to compare filling defects of ^{99m}Tc sulfur colloid with areas of increased ^{123}I antibody uptake. A representative example of such a comparison is shown in figure 3.

This shows the contour of a transverse section of a ^{99m}Tc sulfur colloid liver ECT overlaying the corresponding section of the ^{123}I Mab ECT. The cold area of the sulfur colloid scan representing liver metastases of a right colon carcinoma corresponds to a hot area on the ECT obtained 24 h after intravenous injection of ^{123}I labelled Fab fragments of Mab 35.

The overall sensitivity of tumour detection in our series of 23 patients was rather high. In the 13 patients injected with F(ab')2 fragments labelled with ^{123}I, 23 out of 28 tumour sites were detected by ECT. This includes 6/6 primary or recurrent localized carcinomas, 5/8 patients with liver metastases, 0/2 lung metastases 8 of less than 2 cm diameter and with stable size during a 10 months follow up) and 12/12 bone metastases (in 2 patients). In the 10 patients injected with Fab fragments, 30 out of 31 tumour sites were detected by ECT, including 6/7 primary or recurrent carcinomas, 6/6 patients with liver metastases and 18/18 bone metastases (in a single patient). We realize that this very high sensitivity is due in part to the selection of patients with known tumours and to the relatively large size of the tumours detected. The smallest primary tumour detected was a carcinomatous polyp of the rectum weighing 4.5 g and the smallest liver metastases detected had less than 3 cm in diameter as determined by the CT-scan.

DISCUSSION

The major advantage of the use of tomoscintigraphy and ^{123}I labelled Mab fragment consists in the high quality of the images which allows to distinguish tumour accumulation of radioactivity from physiological organ concentration and circulating radioactivity without the artifacts inherent to the subtraction technique. Our optimistic results in term of sensitivity should be confirmed in a prospective study in order to prove that this type of immunotomoscintigraphy can compete with the most modern morphological diagnostic methods such as CT-scan and nuclear magnetic resonance. In any case, we think that for diagnostic purposes small fragments of Mab with high affinity for a relatively

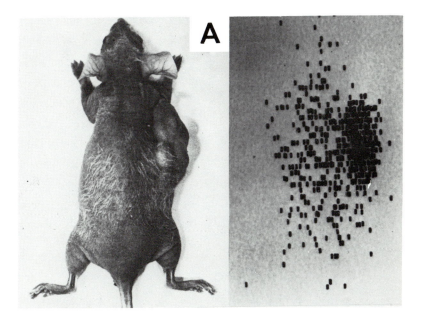

Figure 2: Comparison of the scans of nude mice grafted with human colon carcinoma obtained either 3-days after injection of 131 I-labelled immunoabsorbent purified polyclonal goat anti-CEA antibodies (panel A) or 2 days after injection of 131 I-labelled Fab fragments from monoclonal antibody 35 (panel B). The tumour of the mouse on panel A weighed 1.8 g. whereas the tumour on the mouse on panel B weighed only 0.1 g. tumour.

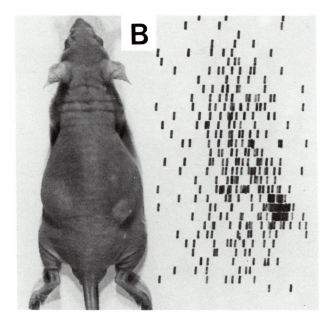

Figure 2 b.

abundant tumour marker such as CEA represent the best tracer. If one considers the use of radiolabelled antibody for therapy, however, the strategy might be different, because of the too rapid renal excretion of the Fab fragments which has only a 50,000 molecular weight.

Only three groups have reported results of radioimmunotherapy. The group of Order (10,18) has used semi-purified polyclonal antibodies against CEA and ferritin, labelled with therapeutic doses of ^{131}I to treat biliary tract carcinoma and hepatoma, respectively. The moderately optimistic results obtained, may be due to the fact that a high percentage of the injected polyclonal antibodies will always accumulate in the liver and therefore may have some usefulness against these two types of liver tumour. Despite great improvement in the dosimetric analysis of the target organ (18) the specificity of the localization in terms of tumour to normal tissue ratios remains difficult to evaluate. Larson et al. (19) have used intact and Fab fragments of Mab directed against the the p-97 melnoma associated antigen in the treatment of this tumour. Despite the repeated injection of relatively high doses (100 mCi) of ^{131}I, the anti-tumour effect has been very modest. Recently, a research group from the Hammersmith Hospital has reported on the intra-peritoneal, -pleural or -pericardial injection of Mab anti-milk fat globule antigen (20), labelled with 20 mCi of ^{131}I, in 3 patients with different types of carcinomas invading these anatomical cavities (21). The remissions observed, however, are not numerous enough to conclude that they are due to the specificity of the injected radiolabelled antibodies.

In conclusion, the detection of human cancer by radiolabelled antibodies has markedly improved, thanks to the Mab selection and fragmentation as well as to the recent advances in nuclear medicine technology. We do not yet know, however, if the tumour uptake of labelled antibodies which are useful for diagnosis may justify the administration of larger amounts of radioactivity bound to Mab for therapy.

REFERENCES

1. Kohler G., Milstein C. Continuous cultures of fused cells secreting antibody of predefined specificity. Nature 1975; 256:495–497.

2. Pressman D., Korngold L. The in vivo localization of anti-Wagner osteogenic sarcoma antibodies. Cancer 1953; 6:619–623.

3. Bale W.F., Spar I.L., Goodland R.L. Wolfe D.E. In vivo and in vitro studies of labelled antibodies against rat kidney and Walker carcinoma. Proc. Soc. Exp. Biol. Med. 1955;89:564–568.

4. Mach J.P. Carrel S., Merenda C., Sordat B., Cerottini J.C. In vivo localization of radiolabelled antibodies to carcinoembryonic antigen in human colon carcinoma grafted into nude mice. Nature 1974; 248:704–706.

5. Goldenberg D.M., Preston D.F., Primus F.J., Hansen H.J. Photoscan localization of GW–39 tumours in hamsters using radiolabelled anti-carcinoembryonic antigen immunoglobulin G. Cancer Res. 1974; 34:1–9.

6. Goldenberg D.M., Deland F., Enishin D., Bennett S., Primus F.J. van Nagell J.R. Estes N., DeSimone P. Rayburn P. Use of radiolabelled antibodies to carcinoembryonic antigen for the detection and localization of diverse cancers by external photoscanning. N. Engl. J. Med. 178; 298:1384–1388.

7. Goldenberg D.M. Kim E.D. Deland F.H., Bennett S., Primus

F.J. Radioimmunodetection of cancer with radioactive antibodies to carcinoembryonic antigen. Cancer Res. 1980; 40:2984-2992.

8. Mach J.P. Carrel S., Forni M., Ritschard J., Donath A., Alberto P. Tumor localization of radiolabelled antibodies against carcinoembryonic antigen in patients with carcinoma. N. Engl. J. Med. 1980; 303:5-10.

9. Mach J.P., Forni M., Ritschard J., Buchegger F., Carrel S., Widgren S., Donath A., Alberto P. Use and limitations of radiolabelled anti-CEA antibodies and their fragments for photoscanning detection of human colorectal carcinomas. (Oncodevelop. Biol. Med. 1980; 1:46-69.

10. Ettinger O., Order S.E. Wharam M.D., Parker M.K. Klein J.L., Keicher P.K. Phase I-II study of isotopic immunoglobulin therapy for primary liver cancer. Cancer Treatment Reports 1982; 66:289-297.

11. Mach. J.P. Buchegger F., Forni M., Ritschard J., Berche C., Lubroso J.D., Schreyer M. Girardet Ch., Accolla R.S. Carrel S. Use of radiolabelled monoclonal anti-CEA antibodies for the detection of human carcinomas by external photoscanning and tomoscintigraphy. Immunology Today 1981; 2:239-249.

12. Accolla R.S., Carrel S., Mach J.P. Monoclonal antibodies specific for carcinoembryonic antigen and rpoduced by two hybrid cell lines. Proc. Natl. Acad. Sci (USA) 1980; 77:563-566.

13. Kuhl D.E. Edwards R.D. Image separation radioisotope scanning. Radiology 1963; 653-662.

14. Berche D., Mach J.P., Lumbroso J.D., Langlais C., Aubry F., Buchegger F., Carrel S., Rouigier P., Parmentier D., Tubiana M. Tomoscintigraphy for detecting gastrointestinal and medullary thyroid cancers : First clinical results using radiolabelled monoclonal antibodies against carcinoembryonic antigen. Brit. Med.

J. 1982; 1447-1451.

15. Haskell C.M., Buchegger F., Schreyer M., Carrel S., Mach J.P. Monoclonal antibodies to carcinoembryonic antigen : ionic strength as a factor in the selection of antibodies for immunoscintigraphy. Cancer Reasearch. (in press).

16. Buchegger F., Schreyer M., Carrel S., Mach J.P. Monoclonal antibody identify a CEA crossreacting antigen of 95 KD (NCA-95) distinct in antigenicity and tissue distribution from the previously described NCA of 55 KD. Int. J. Cancer. 33: 643-649.

17. Buchegger F., Haskell C.M. Schreyer M., Scazziga B.R., Randin S., Carrel S., Mach J.P. Radiolabelled fragments of monoclonal anti-CEA antibodies for localization of human colon carcinoma grafted into nude mice. J. Exp. Med. 1983; 158:413-427.

18. Leichner P.K., Klein J.L., Siegelman S.S., Ettinger D.S., Order S.E., Dosimery of ^{131}I labelled anti-ferritin in hepatoma : Specific activities in the tumor and liver. Cancer Treatment Report 1983; 67.647-658.

19. Larson S.M., Carrasquillo J.A., Krohn K.A. Brown J.P. McGuffin R.W., Ferens J.M., Graham M.M., Hill L.D. Beaumier P.L., Hellstrom K.E., Hellstrom I. Localization of 131-I-labelled p97-specific Fab fragments in human melanoma as a basis for radiotherapy. The Journal of Clinical Investigation 1983; 2101-2114.

20. Granowska M., Shepher J., Britton K.E., Ward B., Mather S., Taylor-Papdimitriou J., Epenetos A.S., Carroll M.J., Nimmon C.C., Hawkins L.A. Slevin M., Flatman W., Horne T., Burchell J., Durbin H. and Bodmer W. Ovarian cancer: diagnosis using ^{131}I monoclonal antibody in comparison with surgical findings. Nuclear Medicine Communications 1983; 5:485-499.

21. Hammersmith Oncology Group and Imperial Cancer Research Fund. Antibody–guided irradiation of malignant lesions: Three cases illustrating a new method of treatment. Lancet 1984. I.1441–1443

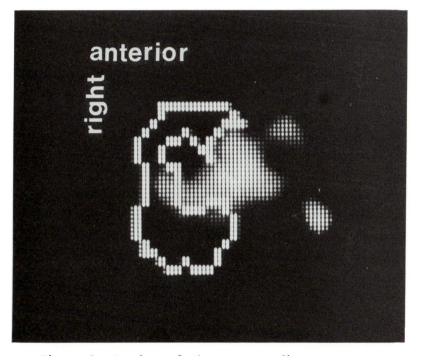

Figure 3: Overlay of the corresponding transverse sections obtained by emission computerized tomography of the liver after injection of 123 I labelled Fab fragments of Mab 35 (dashed area) and 99m Tc labelled sulfur colloid (contour). The 123 I antibody uptake corresponds to the cold area delineated on the 99m Tc sulfur colloid scan.

359

Immunoscintigraphic diagnosis of recurrences of Colorectal cancers. Results compared with those of Ultrasonography and Computed Tomography

Chatal J.F., Saccavini J.C., Douillard J.Y., Kremer M.,
Curtet C., Aubry J. and Le Mevel B.
U.211 INSERM and Centre Rene Gauducheau, Nantes, France.
Office des Rayonnements Ionisants, Saclay, France.

In patients operated on for colorectal carcinoma and having a high risk of recurrence, serial serum assays of tumor markers, namely the carcinoembryonic antigen (CEA) and the CA 19-9 antigen, enable a recurrence to be detected before clinical signs appear. The recurrence must then be confirmed and localized, and its spread determined, to allow the surgeon to decide on his approach if a second resection is feasible. Such is the potential role of immunoscintigraphy after injection of radioiodinated monoclonal antibodies. Initially, a retrospective study enabled the diagnostic sensitivity of the method to be determined as a function of the type of antibodies injected. It also contributed to optimizing the detection parameters. A prospective study was then performed to determine the clinical value of immunoscintigraphy as compared with that of conventional diagnostic methods, that is, ultrasonography and computed tomography.

RETROSPECTIVE STUDY

This study was performed using monoclonal antibodies

designated as 17-1A and 19-9, which were kindly provided by Prof. H. Koprowski, Wistar Institute, Philadelphia, U.S.A. These two antibodies recognize two different antigens associated with gastrointestinal carcinomas. They were labelled with iodine 131 by the iodogen method, with a specific activity of 5 to 10 mCi/mg for intact antibodies and 2 to 5 mCi/mg for $F(ab')_2$ fragments. An activity of 2 to 3 mCi was diluted in 100 ml of saline solution and injected IV during 30 min into each patient. With antibody 17-1A, 54% of tumour sites were visualized (1), whereas the 21 cases of nonepitheliomatous gastrointestinal cancers or nongastrointestinal cancers gave negative results. With antibody 19-9, 66% of tumour sites were visualized (2). For each case studied, regardless of the nature of the antibody, the best contrast of tumour activity to background was obtained more than 4 to 5 days after injection (Fig. 1). It was thus unnecessary to have recourse to the questionable practice of computerized subtraction which can introduce images of artefacts. It may be useful to repeat scans at 2-day intervals to determine whether a poorly contrasted focus is specific or not.

To improve diagnostic sensitivity, it is also possible to inject a combination of antibodies with complementary specificities, such as anti-CEA, 19-9 or 17-1A. An immunohistochemical study, performed with the anti-CEA 202 antibody (kindly provided by Dr. J.P. Mach, Lausanne, Switzerland) and 19-9, demonstrated that some tumours or their recurrences expressed only one of the two antigens and that, when both antigens were expressed, the expression was quantitatively different. It is thus advisable to inject a combination of radioiodinated antibodies, expecially within the scope of a prospective study in which the antigenic expression of the tumour is obviously unknown beforehand.

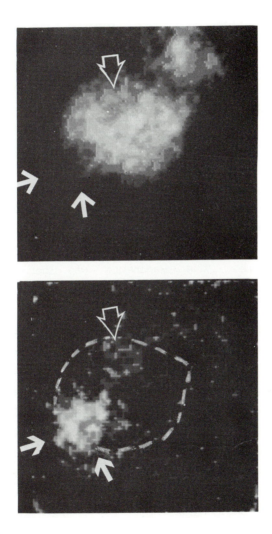

la.

1b.

Fig. 1.

Liver metastasis of colon carcinoma. Immunoscintigraphy performed 5 days after injection of a cocktail of ^{131}I anti-CEA and 19–9 F(ab')2.

1a. ^{99}Tc sulphur colloid liver scan. Anterior view. Photon-deficient areas in the lower (closed arrows) and upper (open arrow) right lobe.

1b. Im munoscintigraphy. Hot spots corresponding to photodeficient areas. Image obtained without computerized subtraction. The outline of the liver is taken from the corresponding ^{99m}Tc image.

PROSPECTIVE STUDY

Immunoscintigraphy was the first examination performed for 25 patients who had undergone surgery for colorectal cancer and were suspected of having a recurrence suggested by clinical and/or biological studies. This examination was then followed by ultrasonography in 19 cases and by computed tomography in 18.

Out of 18 recurrence sites in 16 patients, which were confirmed by surgery or agreement among several diagnostic methods, immunoscintigraphy was positive in 13 cases (72%). Analysis of the comparative results of the three diagnostic methods showed good complementary. For the 19 patients who had immunoscintigraphy and ultrasonography, the results of both examination were in agreement 5 times (3 positive and 2 negative). Ultrasonography was positive in 3 cases of recurrence which were negative with immunoscintigraphy, whereas immunoscintigraphy was positive in 5 cases considered negative with ultrasonography (2 cases of local pelvic recurrence, 2 of abdominal recurrence and 1 of liver metastasis).

For the 18 patients who had immunoscintigraphy and computed tomography the results of both examinations were in agreement 5 times (3 positive and 2 negative). Computed tomography correct a false-negative result of immunoscintigraphy in 2 cases. Finally, computed tomography was negative or doubtful in 7 cases which were positive in immunoscintigraphy. In 4 cases, immunoscintigraphy was the only positive examination and was the basis of the decision to reoperate. In 3 of these cases, the surgeon was able to perform a total resection of the recurrence. In the fourth case, immunoscintigraphy had visualized a pelvic recurrence but not an associated liver recurrence in the form of 2 small metastases each 2 cm in diameter.

On the basis of this preliminary prospective study, it would appear logical to begin assessment of the spread of the desease by immunoscintigraphy using the radiolabelled antibody or antibodies which recognize the antigen with an elevated serum concentration indicate of recurrence. However, the effectiveness of conventional planar scintigraphy is limited by the low ratio of tumour activity to adjacent background.

FUTURE PROSPECTS

Tomoscintigraphy allows an increase in tumour contrast and thus could improve diagnostic sensitivity. However, the low activities of 1 to 2 mCi usually injected require early recording within 2 days after injection to obtain a satisfactory count statistic, in which case interpretation of the images is hampered by the existence of multiple nonspecific Foci (3). In order to reduce the number of contrast of these Foci, and thus to improve the specificity of the method, it is necessary, as for conventional planar scintigraphy, to wait 4 to 5 days after injection, which entails an increase in the activity injected and a lengthening of the recording time. In these conditions, that is, for an activity of 3 to 3.5 mCi and a recording time of 40 min., the count statistic

365

is satisfactory and the image easier to interpret (Fig.2).

Fig. 2   Local recurrence of rectum carcinoma. Pelvic tomoimmunoscintigraphy performed 4 days after injection of a cocktail of ^{131}I anti-CEA and 19-9 F(ab')$_2$.

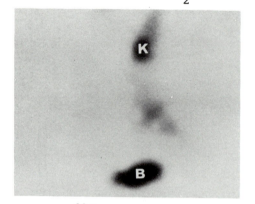

2a Sagittal section ^{99m}Tc HMDP

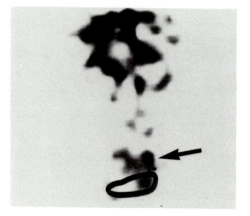

2b. Sagittal section. ^{131}I. Hot spot above the posterior part of the bladder (arrow).

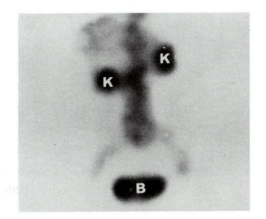

2c. Coronal section. ^{99m}Tc HMDP.

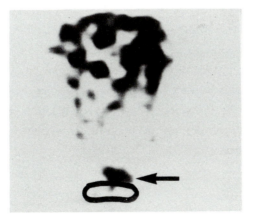

2d. Coronal section. ^{131}I. Hot spot above the left part of the bladder (arrow).

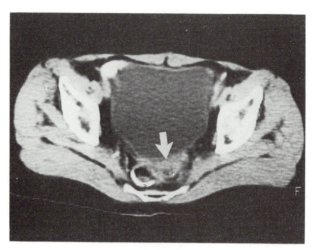

B = Bladder

K = Kidney

2e. CTscan. Mass behind the bladder.

On images 2b and 2d the outline of the bladder is taken from the corresponding ^{99m}Tc images.

CONCLUSION

In order to localize a recurrence of colorectal carcinoma, immunoscintigraphy after injection of a combination of radioiodinated monoclonal antibodies appears to be a useful method which is complementary to those involving a morphological approach such as ultrasonography and computed tomography. The application of tomoscintigraphy should contribute to improving diagnostic sensitivity.

REFERENCES

1. Mach J.P., Chatal J.F., Lumbroso J.D. et al (1983). Cancer Res. 43, 5593-5600.

2. Chatal J.F., Saccavini J.C., Fumoleau P. et al (1984). J. Nucl. Med. 25, 307-314.

3. Mach J.P., Buchegger F., Forni M. et al. (1981). Immunol. Today 2, 239-249.

Radioimmunoscintigraphy of the Lymphatic System versus Intravenous application of Tumour-associated Monoclonal Antibodies: Indications and Clinical usefulness in the management of cancer patients.

Pateisky N.*, Philipp K.*, Skodler D.*, Burchell J.*.

* Department of Obstetrics and Gynaecology,
   University of Vienna.

** Imperial Cancer Research Fund, Lincoln's Inn Fields
   London.

SUMMARY

Radioimmunoscintigraphy provides a very helpful tool in the management of cancer patients. In our study two forms of application using a monoclonal tumor-associated antibody labelled by I-123 were carried out depending on the area investigated. The intravenous route was used to search for ovarian carcinoma and it's metastases, while the subcutaneous route of application seemed to be favourable to investigate lymph nodes in the pathways of different carcinomas.

MATERIALS AND METHODS

The monoclonal tumor-associated antibody HMFG-2 which was used by us was provided by the ICRF-Laboratories (London) and reacts strongly with malignant cells of epithelian origin. Radioactive labelling with I-123 was done by the IODOGEN-method (1). The production of the antibody is described elsewhere (2). After the labelling-procedure the radioantibody was given to the patients intravenously or subcutaneously respectively, in a dose between 1,5 and 2 mCi. The specific activity of the labelled antibodies ranged between 2 and 5 mCi/mg antibody. Static scintigrams accumulated up to 300.000 count were then made up to 24 hours after injection of the radioantibody. Most of the patients were operated on a few days after the scanning-procedure, so that the operation sites could be compared with the findings on the Immunoscintigram.

RESULTS

Two groups of patients were investigated by the method of Radioimmunoscintigraphy to estimate the clinical usefulness of the two methods of administration (i.v., s.c.).

The 15 patients in the first group were all women with the suspicion of malignant ovarian tumours or recurrent disease of ovarian carcinoma (Table 1). In four out of the 10 patients with a known history of ovarian carcinoma, tumour sites could be revealed by Immunoscintigraphy which could not be detected by any other investigative method. In these four patients further therapy could be initiated at an optimal time. In 3 of the patients a second look operation and in 1 patient irradiation therapy were performed.

Table 1

	pos (n=12)		neg (n=3)
correct	false	correct	false
11	1	2	1

Scan results of patients with suspicion of having ovarian carcinoma or recurrent desease.

The second group included 7 patients with x-ray confirmed breast carcinoma. Prior to the operation Radioimmunolymphscans (3) of both the axillary lymphatics of the affected as well as the nodes of the healthy side were carried out and compared with the histological report of the surgical removed lymph nodes. Table two shows an overview of the confirmed scan results of the lymphatics of the affected side. All scan results of the healthy side were negative.

Table 2

	pos (4)		neg (3)
correct	false	correct	false
3	1	2	1

Scan results of axillary lymphatics in patients with breast carcinoma.

CONCLUSION

Radioimmunoscintigraphy turns out to be of considerable help in the management of ovarian carcinoma using the technique of intravenous administration of radioantibody. Especially in the follow up of patients with a known history of ovarian carcinoma, tumour sites can be detected which may not be diagnosed by any other method.

Although the number of patients investigated by Radiolymph immunoscintigraphy is too small to give a final judgement, there seems to be some hope for the future in lymph node staging prior to cancer therapy.

Involvement of the method in "Intraoperative Lymph Scintigraphy" (4) could help to improve the radicality of lymphadenectomy during the operative treatment of genaecological malignancies of the cervix, ovary and endometrium, and breast cancer.

REFERENCES

1. Salacinski P., Hope J., McLean C., et al

A New simple method which allows theoretical incorporation of radioiodine into proteins and peptides without damage.

Proc. Soc. Endocrinol. p 131 (1980).

2. Taylor-Papadimitriou J., Peterson J.A., Arklie J. et al

Monoclonal Antibodies to Epithelium-Specific Components of the Human Milk Fat Globule Membrane: Production and Reaction with Cells in Culture.

Int. J. Cancer: 28, 17-21 (1981).

3. Weinstein J.N., Steller M.A., Keenan A.M. et al

Monoclonal Antibodies in the Lymphatics: Selective Delivery to Lymph Node Metastases of a Solid Tumor

Science Vol 222, p.423-426 (1983).

4. Gitsch E., Philipp K., Pateisky N.

Intraoperative Lymph Scintigraphy during Radical Surgery for Cervical Cancer

J. Nucl. Med. 25:486-489, (1984).